# Clinical Management of Memory Problems

## Second edition

Edited by

*Barbara Wilson*

Senior Scientist
MRC Applied Psychology Unit
Cambridge

and

*Nick Moffat*

Top Grade Psychologist
Branksome Clinic
Poole
Dorset

**CHAPMAN & HAL**

London · Glasgow · New York · Tokyo · 

D0353512

**Published by Chapman & Hall, 2–6 Boundary Row, London SE1 8HN**

Chapman & Hall, 2–6 Boundary Row, London SE1 8HN, UK

Blackie Academic & Professional, Wester Cleddens Road, Bishopbriggs, Glasgow G64 2NZ, UK

Chapman & Hall, 29 West 35th Street, New York, NY 10001, USA

Chapman & Hall Japan, Thomson Publishing Japan, Hirakawacho Nemoto Building, 6F, 1–7–11 Hirakawa-cho, Chiyoda-ku, Tokyo 102, Japan

Chapman & Hall Australia, Thomas Nelson Australia, 102 Dodds Street, South Melbourne, Victoria, 3205, Australia

Chapman & Hall India, R. Seshadri, 32 Second Main Road, CIT East, Madras 600 035, India

Distributed in the USA and Canada by Singular Publishing Group Inc., 4284 41st Street, San Diego, California 92105

First edition 1984

Second edition 1992

© 1984, Barbara Wilson and Nick Moffat, 1992 Chapman & Hall

Typeset in 10 on 12pt Palatino by
Falcon Typographic Art Ltd, Fife, Scotland
Printed in Great Britain by
St Edmundsbury Press, Bury St Edmunds, Suffolk

ISBN 0 412 32250 1

A catalogue record for this book is available from the British Library

# Contents

# Contributors

**Alan D. Baddeley**, Director, Medical Research Council Applied Psychology Unit, 15 Chaucer Road, Cambridge.

**Neil Brooks**, Professor of Clinical Psychology, University of Glasgow, Department of Psychological Medicine, 6 Whittinghame Gardens, Great Western Road, Glasgow.

**John Harris**, Proprietor of Cambit, 1 Rowan Close, Bottisham, Cambridge.

**Michael Kopelman**, Senior Lecturer, Academic Department of Psychiatry, United Medical and Dental School, St Thomas's Hospital, Lambeth Palace Road, London.

**Nadina B. Lincoln**, Research Clinical Psychologist, The Stroke Research Unit, The General Hospital, Park Row, Nottingham.

**Nick Moffat**, Top Grade Clinical Psychologist, District Psychology Service, Branksome Clinic, Layton Road, Parkstone, Poole, Dorset.

**Ian Robertson**, Senior Scientist, MRC Applied Psychology Unit, 15 Chaucer Road, Cambridge.

**Clive Skilbeck**, District Clinical Psychologist, Newcastle Health Authority, Royal Victoria Infirmary, Newcastle upon Tyne.

**Deborah Wearing**, Development Manager, AMI, Grafton Manor, Grafton Regis, Towcester, Northampton.

**Barbara Wilson**, Senior Scientist, MRC Applied Psychology Unit, 15 Chaucer Road, Cambridge.

**Rodger Llewellyn-Wood**, Consultant Neuropsychologist, St George's House, 56 Billing Road, Northampton.

# Preface

Since the first edition of this book appeared in 1984, assistance for memory-impaired people has improved a little. The Amnesia Association was founded in 1986 and a number of local Amnass groups meet regularly throughout the United Kingdom. Although help is still hard to find for most patients and their carers, it is now probably a little easier for some memory-impaired people and their families to obtain advice that might enable them to come to terms with the problematic changes that take place in their lives. What is certain is that interest in the rehabilitation of memory problems continues to grow, and this has led to further developments in memory therapy in recent years. The second edition of this book has been compiled in response to this growth of interest and reflects the latest developments and debates within the field of memory therapy.

Memory problems are common after such conditions as severe head injury, progressive degenerative disease, cerebral vascular accident (stroke), chronic alcohol abuse, intracranial infection and certain other conditions. Although this list means that vast numbers of people throughout the world suffer from varying levels of memory impairment, their predicament is largely ignored and remains untreated. It is hoped that this book will stimulate greater interest in their problems and at the same time offer ideas for treatment.

The commonly observed advertisements in the press offering to improve memory are of no practical use whatsoever for the great majority of brain-injured people, who need a protective environment and assistance from competent workers in the field of rehabilitation. Most speech therapists, occupational therapists, clinical psychologists, social workers, doctors, nurses, teachers and physiotherapists are given little guidance as to what methods are available or which methods are suitable for helping individual patients to cope with their memory problems. We said in the first edition that therapists who turn to previous publications on memory were unlikely to obtain much in the way of relevant or practically useful information. Fortunately the situation has improved here as more text books on memory are beginning to address the question of management of memory problems. However, this book remains the only comprehensive guidebook for those working with memory-impaired people. In 1991, as in 1984, we do not provide medical solutions, easy answers or make promises about restoring memory, but we do attempt to give a better understanding of the difficulties faced by people with memory problems and we offer suggestions on how to handle, by-pass or reduce memory difficulties.

Alan Baddeley's chapter serves as an important foundation for the rest of the book in that it describes the fundamental relationship between theory and practice as far as memory and memory therapy are concerned. A clear account of the psychological structure of human memory is provided by the author who himself has done more than anybody else to ensure that there is a thriving two-way communication between theory and therapy in the field of memory rehabilitation.

Before beginning any remediation of memory impairment, an appropriate assessment of the nature of that impairment is required. In Chapter 2 Nadina Lincoln and Neil Brooks describe procedures for carrying out such an assessment. The emphasis is on assessment for rehabilitation rather than for research purposes or for routine administration of tests. The chapter indicates that assessment for rehabilitation is inseparable from treatment and that in order to evaluate the effectiveness of treatment it is necessary to carry out assessment of treatment outcome. The chapter discusses reasons why assessments should occur, who should assess, and when assessments should be made. The authors also include descriptions of some new tests not available in the first edition.

In Chapter 3 John Harris describes methods for improving memory that were available at the time of writing this chapter. He discusses internal strategies, repetitive practice, physical treatments and external aids. Because of the rapid development of some computerized external aids, however, Harris recognizes that some of this chapter will inevitably be out of date by the time the book is published. Harris provides explanations of ways in which various methods seem to work, and offers his own views on their respective strengths and weaknesses.

Nick Moffat begins Chapter 4 with a consideration of variables which may affect memory performance and then discusses the organization of memory therapy. Moffat explains in detail the application of reality orientation training and discusses several methods for improving memory previously described by Harris, examining these within the context of rehabilitation of brain-injured people. Moffat describes a number of recent memory rehabilitation studies reflecting the interest in this topic since the first book appeared.

In Chapter 5, Barbara Wilson discusses memory therapy in practice. She provides some general principles for helping memory impaired people to encode, store and retrieve information before going on to examine specific strategies for particular problems. She discusses ways of teaching memory-impaired people to use strategies, and points out that it is unrealistic to expect most memory-impaired people to use these strategies spontaneously. It is the therapists, relatives and carers who use strategies to help memory-impaired people learn.

When this book first appeared in 1984, microcomputers in rehabilitation were fairly new. In 1991 they are very much in evidence in most rehabilitation programmes. In Chapter 6 Clive Skilbeck and Ian Robertson discuss the advantages and disadvantages of microcomputers, and provide a summary of studies evaluating the use of computers in rehabilitation. The authors suggest that microcomputers should not be expected to restore or significantly improve memory functioning in and of themselves. They should be regarded, rather, as adjuncts to treatment programmes.

Chapter 7 by Michael Kopelman, on the psychopharmacology of human memory disorders, replaces Steven Cooper's chapter on drug treatments, neurochemical change and human memory impairment that appeared in the first edition. Kopelman discusses Korsakoff's syndrome, Alzheimer-type dementia and Huntington's disease. He also reviews studies of the effects of agents modulating neurotransmitter systems in healthy subjects and clinical trials of 'replacement' therapy in amnesic or dementing patients before concluding that most benefits seem to be small and fickle and of little clinical importance.

Attention and speed of information processing are often compromised after brain injury, and in Chapter 8 Rodger Wood considers disorders of attention, alertness, selectivity, effort and memory. He refers the reader to several studies which attempt to identify processes involved in the operation of these skills. During rehabilitation a patient will have to revert to a more conscious and controlled form of information processing, and the second half of the chapter concentrates on various ideas, suggestions and tasks for developing attention-training programmes.

Memory impaired people may benefit from interactions with others sharing similar disabilities. In Chapter 9 Wilson and Moffat discuss several possible advantages to be gained from treating memory-impaired people in groups. Descriptions are provided of group therapy for in-patients, most of whom are young and who have had a severe head injury, and for out-patients with mixed ages and aetiologies. Perhaps the major benefit of memory group therapy is that it reduces anxiety and negative emotions associated with memory impairment rather than improving memory *per se*. Another advantage of groups, perhaps, is that brain-injured people may be more willing to use compensatory strategies if they see their peers using them.

The final chapter of this second edition was not included in the first. It is written by Deborah Wearing, the wife of Clive Wearing, a musician who became densely amnesic in 1985 following herpes simplex encephalitis. Deborah Wearing is co-founder of the Amnesia Association and did a great deal to bring the plight of amnesic patients to the attention of the general public. Her chapter is on self-help groups and is written from a relative's point of view. At the end of the day relatives bear the brunt of coping with a memory-impaired person. For this reason we would encourage all professionals involved in brain-injury rehabilitation to work closely with relatives in order to increase their understanding of the day-to-day problems encountered by memory-impaired people and their families.

# Chapter 1

# Memory theory and memory therapy

## ALAN D. BADDELEY

The present chapter began life as a paper presented at a workshop on memory retraining. The workshop sprang from discussions between research workers primarily concerned with the theoretical understanding of human memory, and practical clinicians concerned with the task of helping particular patients cope with their memory problems. Given such origins, it seemed sensible to begin with a consideration of current theories of memory, and then go on to discuss their application in practice – and I agreed to give the theoretical introduction. I did so, presenting an overview of current approaches to human memory. Having given it, I had very mixed feelings. On the one hand I felt I had made a reasonably competent attempt at the difficult job of surveying the vast amount of research that has gone on in the area of human memory over the last decade. I believe this to be an intrinsically interesting area, and one which is at least of background relevance to anyone working with patients suffering from memory problems. On the other hand, I felt that I had completely fudged the issue of how and why such theoretical research is relevant to the therapist trying to help an individual patient.

The task I avoided was a difficult one, not least because I knew so little of the characteristics of the audience I was addressing, or of the practical problems of memory therapy. Even with the benefit of hindsight, writing about the relationship between theory and practice in an area as new and diverse as this presents substantial problems. I do however believe that it is extremely important to maintain strong and healthy links between theory and practice. What follows attempts to explain why.

THEORY AND PRACTICE

It is sometimes claimed that 'there is nothing so practical as a good theory', a comforting adage for the academic, but is it justified? There is no doubt that in some situations a really good theory can be extremely useful. Let us take a very obvious case such as the role of Newtonian mechanics in structural engineering. It is inconceivable that a structural engineer's education these days would not include an understanding of mechanics. So much so that it is easy to forget that the concepts underlying this are essentially theoretical in nature. A theory is like a map that can help you understand where you are and help you get from one place to another. Scientific theories can be helpful but are not essential; one can find one's way across country without recourse to a map given enough experience, and people were of course building bridges using techniques that were consistent with Newtonian mechanics long before Newton produced his theory.

Like a map, a theory can be useful but requires intelligent interpretation. A theory is not like a recipe giving you a list of things to do in order to achieve a particular aim, although recipe books may in time develop from a theoretical understanding of the field. To go back to our bridge-building, a treatise on mechanics would not tell you how to build a bridge, although it might contain a great deal of extremely useful material if properly applied.    What then can the practising clinician expect to get from theories of memory? I would suggest three things, a general orientation and understanding, suggestions as to particular therapeutic techniques, and finally methodological help in evaluating such techniques.

A THEORETICAL OVERVIEW

While a good therapist will always be aware of the particular characteristics of each individual patient, if he or she is to learn from experience, then it is essential to be aware of what different cases have in common. A good theory, like a map, provides suitable landmarks for identifying where you are at present and helping you reach a specified goal. Consider for example the question of diagnosis; one of the clearest cases of global amnesia due to brain damage that I myself have encountered was a woman who had attempted suicide though coal-gas poisoning. She had the classic amnesia combination of normal immediate memory coupled with a grossly impaired ability to learn new material. She was for some time categorized as a hysteric amnesic simply because her particular pattern of symptoms was inconsistent with her psychiatrist's totally incorrect concept of the structure and breakdown of human memory. In the absence of explicit theory, we all tend to apply our own implicit theories, which can be all the more dangerous for being applied unthinkingly.

## THEORIES AND STRATEGIES

A second way in which theoretical work can be useful is in suggesting new approaches to practical problems. The whole area of behaviour modification in clinical psychology is an offshoot of theoretical approaches to the study of learning, initially in animals. Although the area of memory therapy is still in its infancy, there are already many obvious examples of borrowing techniques devised, or at least explored in the laboratory. These will be discussed in more detail subsequently (Chapters 4 and 5), but examples include distribution of practice, and the manipulation of coding during learning by such strategies as the use of visual imagery and encouraging deep rather than shallow processing.

## EVALUATION OF TECHNIQUES

In the case of memory therapy, this is an area of future importance rather than current achievement. Until techniques are developed and explored, they are obviously not suitable for evaluation. It is however essential that such evaluation does take place. Brain-damaged patients tend to recover spontaneously, and the observation that patients enjoy a particular therapeutic procedure and appear to improve is not by any means an adequate justification for continuing that procedure. The appropriate question is whether such improvement would have occurred anyhow, and if not whether the amount and generality of the improvement is sufficient to justify that degree of expenditure of therapists' and patients' time.

Evaluating the success of memory therapy is likely to prove difficult since it is of course important not to assume that the improvement of patients on laboratory tests of memory will necessarily generalize to everyday memory tasks. However academic psychologists are increasingly aware of the need to study memory outside the laboratory, and should provide potentially useful allies in tackling this difficult problem. The development of the Rivermead Behavioural Memory Test, described in Chapter 5 is a good example of the blending of the experimental control of the laboratory with the richness of the everyday world to provide a test that is both sensitive and realistic.

Most laboratory studies of memory use procedures in which a comparison is made between two or more large groups of similar subjects. The therapist on the other hand is often confronted with the problem of evaluating a technique based on a relatively small number of subjects with widely differing problems. It seems probable that the single case approach to the evaluation of therapy will prove most useful here. The technique, which was originally developed in the animal laboratory by psychologists influenced by the techniques of B. F. Skinner, has been subsequently applied most effectively to the evaluation of treatment methods in connection with behaviour modification (Hersen and Barlow, 1976), but has subsequently been applied very successfully to the treatment of memory problems, most notably by Wilson (1987a, 1987b).

In this chapter I will be primarily concerned with the first two applications of memory theory, namely the provision of an overview together with the suggestion of possible strategies, although these will not be described in any detail since they are covered in Chapters 3, 4 and 5. It goes without saying, however, that if the field is to develop, then the application of new strategies should go hand-in-hand with their evaluation.

## AN OVERVIEW OF HUMAN MEMORY

Suppose a therapist were to accept what I have just argued, and attempt to obtain an overview of current theories of memory, what should he or she do? Start reading current memory journals perhaps? This would be, I suspect, a puzzling and rather dispiriting experience. Journals, and indeed often textbooks, are primarily concerned with points of disagreement and tend to give the bewildering view of any field that it comprises far more controversy than agreement. The reason for this is obvious; people do not write papers about what everyone agrees about, and what is already established does not require further experimentation. However, beneath the controversies and disagreements there is a surprisingly large amount of common ground. The present section will attempt to summarize this and link it to the specific problem of memory therapy. Any overview as brief as this however is inevitably fragmentary. A more extensive account of current views of memory for the non-specialist is given in Baddeley (1982a).

## HOW MANY KINDS OF MEMORY?

This is a question that has preoccupied psychologists quite extensively over the last 30 years. It has been, and remains, an area of controversy. The non-specialist attempting to understand this area is likely to be puzzled not only by theoretical differences between different authorities, but also by a wide range of different terms often used to refer to very similar concepts. However, since I myself would regard the conceptual distinctions underlying this controversial area as being very important in evaluating and understanding memory breakdown, I shall discuss the area in some detail.

In talking about remembering or forgetting, we tend to refer to 'my memory', as if it were a single organ like the heart or liver. Over the last 20 years, however, it has become increasingly obvious that memory does not represent a single system, but is rather a complex combination of memory subsystems. The available evidence argues very strongly against the idea of a single unitary organ. Some psychologists still argue for what they describe as a unitary system, but when looked at in detail it is a system of such complexity that it could equally well be described as a multiple memory system. To revert to our analogy of theories as maps, it is as if early cartographers were arguing about whether Europe, Asia and Africa should be regarded as one continent or several. What follows represents a simplification of some complex issues. However, although I am sure my colleagues would disagree in detail, there would I think be broad agreement on the functional distinctions underlying the classification system described.

I shall begin by dividing memory into three categories, broadly based on the length of time for which they store information. The division was probably expressed most clearly by Atkinson and Shiffrin, and is presented most convincingly for the general reader in their *Scientific American* article (Atkinson and Shiffrin, 1971). They assume a very brief set of sensory stores, followed by a limited capacity short-term store which in turn feeds information into a long-term memory store. In what follows we shall use this as a framework, while pointing out the ways in which the Atkinson and Shiffrin model has proved to be oversimplified.

## SENSORY MEMORY

The various sensory systems such as vision, audition and touch are all assumed to be capable of storing sensory information for a brief period of time. The most extensively investigated component of this system is the very short-term visual store sometimes known as *iconic memory*. It is this system that makes cinematography possible. A series of separate and discrete still pictures, each separated by a blank period is perceived as a single moving figure since the information is stored during the blank interval and integrated into a single percept. In the case of the auditory system a very brief sensory store sometimes termed *echoic memory* allows us to perceive speech sounds. In the case of both vision and hearing, the systems are relatively complex, almost certainly involving more than a single sensory memory trace. A breakdown in such a system would however almost certainly manifest itself as a perceptual difficulty rather than a memory problem, and as such is beyond the scope of the present chapter.

## SHORT-TERM WORKING MEMORY

The second system described by Atkinson and Shiffrin is one which they refer to as the short-term store or STS. They assume this system to be responsible for temporarily holding information while learning, reading, reasoning or thinking. They assume a distinction between this and a long-term memory system – the long-term store (LTS) which preserves information for anything ranging from minutes to years.

The distinction between these two systems, LTS and STS, evoked a great deal of controversy during the late 1960s and early 1970s. This particularly concerned the question of whether it was necessary to assume a separate temporary or short-term storage system. Anyone attempting to read about this particular controversy should be warned of two pitfalls connected with the term 'short-term memory'. The first of these is to be aware of the fact that experimental psychologists use this term to refer to memory extending typically over a few seconds only. This is potentially very misleading since the public in general, and many medical practioners, tend to use the term to refer to memory extending over minutes, days, weeks or months, reserving the term 'long-term memory' for memory for events happening many years before. The available experimental evidence suggests that the most appropriate temporal distinction occurs between a few seconds and a few minutes. Nevertheless the term short-term memory is clearly potentially highly misleading and hence will not be used subsequently in this chapter. Other terms that have been suggested in place of short-term memory include **primary memory** (with long-term memory being referred to as **secondary memory**), **immediate memory** and **working memory**. I will use the term primary memory to refer to the simple concept of a unitary temporary memory system such as that suggested by Atkinson and Shiffrin, and will employ the term working memory to refer to a subsequent view, namely that we utilize a whole range of interacting temporary storage systems rather than a single primary memory.

We shall begin by briefly considering the evidence for separating primary and secondary memory, then present the evidence for a complex working memory rather than a simple primary memory system before going on to a more detailed consideration of long-term memory. Evidence that prompted people to distinguish primary and secondary memory in the late 1960s included the following:

### Tasks with two components

A number of memory tests behave as though they are determined by two separate sets of factors. Consider for example the task known as *free recall* in which subjects see or hear a list of about 20 unrelated words which they must subsequently try to recall in any order they wish. Figure 1.1 shows the typical performance of a subject on this task; the vertical axis indicates the probability of recalling a particular word and the horizontal axis the order in which the words were presented. Note that when recalled immediately, the first few words are quite well recalled and the last few very well. If instead of allowing subjects to recall straightaway, however, one delays them for 15 or 20 seconds, meanwhile preventing them rehearsing the words by giving another task such as copying letters, one obtains the results shown in the delayed recall curve of Figure 1.1 (Postman and Phillips, 1965). The advantage previously enjoyed by the last few items, known as the *recency effect* since these are the most recent items, disappears. In contrast, performance on the earlier items is unaffected.

One way of explaining this result is to suggest that all items are registered in a relatively durable secondary or long-term memory store, but that only the last few items are held in a temporary primary memory system. If recall is delayed, the items in the primary memory system are forgotten leaving only the contents of the more durable secondary store. Other evidence in favour of this distinction comes from the fact that a great many factors that influence the ease of remembering the earlier items have no effect on recency. These include the rate at which the words are presented (slow presentation leads to better recall), the familiarity of the words (familiar words are easier), whether the words are

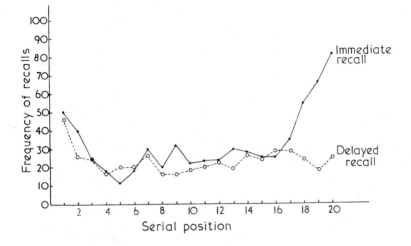

**Figure 1.1** The effective delay on the free recall of words (data from Postman and Phillips, 1965).

concrete and imageable (imageability helps learning) and so forth. None of these factors influences the recency effect, which is however very sensitive to delay.

If one considers not the material but the people learning the material, then again a clear distinction appears between performance on the recency items and performance on the remainder. This shows up most strikingly in Figure 1.2 which is based on a study comparing globally amnesic patients with control patients having normal memory. Note that performance over the recency part of the curve is equivalent in the two groups, whereas performance on the earlier long-term items is much poorer in the amnesic patients.

### Evidence from amnesia

As Figure 1.2 shows, patients occur who appear to have normal primary memory as measured by the recency effect in free recall, coupled with disastrously poor long-term or secondary memory. This distinction is not limited to free recall. Such patients have normal digit span, that is they can repeat back a sequence of numbers they have just heard just as effectively as could control patients. They may also have intact performance on the short-term forgetting task devised by Peterson and Peterson (1959), although this task is a demanding one which is not always intact in amnesic patients, particularly if they have cognitive deficits that go beyond a pure memory problem (see Baddeley, 1982b for a further discussion of this point).

Not only does one find certain patients who have normal primary memory coupled with impaired long-term or secondary memory, but one also encounters cases where the reverse applies. Shallice and Warrington (1970) describe a patient who shows normal long-term learning coupled with grossly defective primary memory as measured by digit span or by the recency effect in free recall. A number of other cases showing a broadly similar pattern of normal long-term coupled with impaired primary memory have been described and present a strong case for separating the two memory systems (for a further discussion see Baddeley (1982c) and Shallice (1979)).

*Coding and memory*

If subjects are given a sequence of unrelated words and required to repeat them back immediately, they will tend to remember them in terms of their sound or articulatory characteristics. If the words are similar along this dimension (e.g. *man, cat, map, can*), the items are liable to become confused in memory leading to more errors than would be found with a dissimilar sequence (e.g. *pen, day, rig, cow, bar*) (Baddeley, 1966a). In contrast, if subjects are required to learn a longer sequence of words, and are prevented from saying them immediately by interposing a delay, other factors become important. Spoken similarity ceases to be a significant variable, but similarity of meaning becomes important. Hence a sequence comprising adjectives of similar meaning such as *big, long, huge, great, tall* etc. would create more problems than a sequence of dissimilar adjectives such as *old, late, thin, hot, wild* etc., despite the fact that similarity of meaning does not appear to influence immediate recall (Baddeley, 1966b).

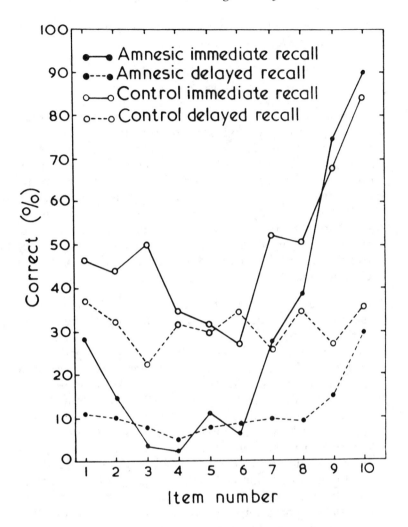

**Figure 1.2** Immediate and delayed recall of words by amnesic and control patients (data from Baddeley and Warrington, 1970).

The initial suggestion was that the primary or short-term system relies on some form of speech code whereas long-term memory relies more extensively on meaning. While this proved to be an over-simplification, as we shall see later there is an interesting and important relationship between the manner in which a subject encodes or processes an item and how well it is remembered.

The original concept of a short-term or primary memory system proposed by Atkinson and Shiffrin treated it as a unitary component. They assumed that information entered the secondary long-term system via the primary short-term store. It was assumed that material was maintained in the temporary storage system, primarily by subvocal rehearsal, and that the longer it was held in the short-term system the greater the chance that it would be transferred to the more durable long-term memory store. However, a number of results emerged that cast doubt on this. These included the following:

1. A number of experiments had been carried out in which subjects were required to continually repeat items. The Atkinson and Shiffrin model predicted that the longer the repetition went on, the better the learning. No relationship between rehearsal time and amount learnt was observed in several of these studies (e.g. Craik and Watkins, 1973).
2. If the recency effect in free recall is due to primary memory, and if the primary memory system can hold only a small amount of material, then giving the subject another primary memory task to do at the same time as learning should wipe out the recency effect. Baddeley and Hitch (1974) showed that giving subjects a telephone number to remember at the same time as they were hearing unrelated words impaired their long-term learning, but had no effect on recency.
3. If the primary memory system is essential for long-term learning, then any patient with a defective primary memory should show grossly impaired long-term learning. As we saw in the case of the patient discussed by Shallice and Warrington (1970) this was not the case.

These and a range of other findings convinced Graham Hitch and me that we should abandon the idea of a single unitary primary memory system and opt instead for the concept of **working memory**. This is assumed to be an alliance of temporary storage systems co-ordinated by an attentional component which we term the **central executive**.

The central executive is assumed to be able to call on a number of subsidiary slave systems. Two such systems have been explored in some detail, namely the articulatory loop and the visuospatial sketch pad. The articulatory loop is a system that utilizes subvocal speech and that is responsible for the speech-like characteristics of many short-term memory tasks. The visuospatial sketch pad is a temporary system used in creating and manipulating visual images. A more detailed analysis of the type of patient discussed by Shallice and Warrington suggests that the crucial deficit is in the short-term phonological store (Vallar and Baddeley, 1984). More recent studies have indicated that patients with a deficit in this system may have problems in comprehending complex sentences (Baddeley, Vallar and Wilson, 1987), and may also find new phonological learning very difficult (Baddeley, Papagno and Vallar, 1988). Since a deficit in short-term phonological memory is probably common in aphasic patients, it suggests that phonological relearning may also be defective, implying that further investigation of this aspect of working memory may well prove important for speech therapy.

The visuospatial sketch pad probably plays an important role in the perception and processing of spatial information. It is almost certainly the case that neuropsychological deficits in this system do occur (Farah, 1988), and have implications for therapy. However, our understanding of this system is still at a relatively early stage.

Working memory is able to utilize a range of parallel subsidiary systems, and it seems likely that a defect in any single one of these may not prove too catastrophic; hence the ability of Shallice and Warrington's patient to show normal long-term learning of meaningful material despite grossly impaired primary memory as measured by digit span. In contrast, a failure of the central executive would be likely to limit very severely the patient's ability to process information and to cope with everyday living. Techniques for identifying a defect of the central executive are still in their infancy (Baddeley, 1986). However it has been suggested (Rabbitt, 1981; Welford, 1980) that the decrement in performance found with advancing age may reflect a deterioration in working memory. The even more dramatic degradation that occurs in the case of presenile and senile dementia may represent a more serious breakdown in the central executive.

One assumed function of the central executive is to co-ordinate tasks involving two or more concurrent sources of information. This was studied in Alzheimer patients and in normal controls of the same age. Subjects were required simultaneously to perform two tasks, one involving immediate memory for numbers, while the other was a motor task involving following a moving light with a pointer. Both of these tasks were adjusted in difficulty for each subject to a point at which all subjects were performing at an equal error rate when the tasks were performed singly. When required to perform both tasks at the same time however, the Alzheimer patients deteriorated to a much greater extent than the normal elderly, a result that supports the view that such patients may have a particular deficit in the central executive component of working memory (Baddeley, Logie, Bressi, Della Sala and Spinnler, 1986).

LONG-TERM OR SECONDARY MEMORY

Most patients referred for treatment of memory problems are likely to be suffering from some form of long-term or secondary memory defect. Such patients are likely to show impaired learning whether this is tested within a few minutes of learning or is delayed for several days or even weeks. As mentioned earlier, the system of memory responsible for retaining information over minutes appears to be broadly the same as that involved in remembering items over a much longer period. However, this does not mean that even the long-term memory constitutes a single unitary system. Two distinctions will be discussed, one a relatively simple division between visual and verbal memory, and the other a more subtle distinction between episodic memory and semantic memory or memory for knowledge.

## VISUAL AND VERBAL MEMORY

If a normal person is shown a series of pictures of easily nameable objects, and subsequently tries to recall them, there is evidence to suggest that his memory will be based on two features of the objects, their visual appearance and their names. This being so, memory tends to be better for such pictures than it would have been purely for their names, since nameable pictures are often represented in two ways, visual and verbal, while words are more likely to be represented in only one. At a common sense level, it is clear that we can remember both things that we can name, and things that we cannot adequately describe verbally, for example, the colour of a particular sunset or the characteristic smile of a friend. This distinction can be very important clinically, since visual and verbal processing tend to be associated with different parts of the brain, and hence one may be disrupted while the other is intact.

From a practical viewpoint this means that it is always important if dealing with patients with defective memory to test both their verbal and visual capabilities. If one is relatively preserved then this can be used to help compensate for the defective aspect of memory. For example, if a subject has verbal memory difficulties but has good visual memory, then visual imagery may provide a useful supplement to normal learning strategies (Jones, 1974; Wilson, 1982). If on the other hand visual memory is grossly defective, then visual imagery would obviously not be the strategy of choice (see Chapter 5).

## SEMANTIC AND EPISODIC MEMORY

The term *semantic memory* is used to refer to memory for knowledge. Remembering the name of the capital of the USA, the French word for salt or the approximate population of Great Britain would be examples of semantic memory. Typically, one cannot remember the occasion on which a particular item of semantic information was learned, usually because learning has taken place over many and varied occasions. This can be contrasted with **episodic memory** which is much more autobiographical in nature. Remembering what you had for breakfast or recalling an incident that occurred on holiday last year would be examples of episodic memory. Recall in this case typically requires awareness of the specific learning incident rather than access to general knowledge. Clearly, most memory situations have components of both semantic and episodic memory. Remembering what you had for breakfast is likely to be at least partially dependent on knowledge of your general breakfast habits as well as recollection of a particular event. It also seems likely that items that are now in semantic memory were first represented as individual episodes. Consider for example the French word for 'salt'; this was probably first told to you in a French lesson at school. If you were questioned about it that evening, then attempting to recall it would almost certainly have relied on episodic memory. By now, if you remember it at all, it seems likely that it is as a result of a wide range of subsequent episodes which you can probably no longer recall.

If most situations represent a blend of semantic and episodic memory, is the distinction worth making? It probably is for two reasons; first, because the ways in which the two systems behave appear to be different, and secondly because certain amnesic patients appear to show a breakdown in episodic memory while showing relatively intact semantic memory. Most of the work carried out on learning by psychologists has been concerned with episodic memory since it is much quicker and easier to study than semantic memory. If the distinction between the two is justified, then we should be wary of generalizing our results too indiscriminately.

There is no doubt that patients may be densely amnesic, and yet perform normally on tests of semantic memory. However, such tests typically test the retention of information about the language and the world that has been learned very thoroughly, typically, many years prior to the onset of amnesia. There is some evidence to suggest that well-learned episodes of a similar age are also well preserved. Furthermore adding new material to semantic memory appears to be just as hard for amnesic patients as new episodic learning. Hence, although semantic memory can be well preserved in some patients, the evidence does not argue strongly for neurologically distinct semantic and episodic memory systems (see Wilson and Baddeley, 1988, for a more detailed discussion).

## PROCEDURAL AND DECLARATIVE LEARNING

There is however evidence that one type of learning, sometimes termed *procedural learning*, may be intact in amnesic patients. Consider in more detail the case of certain amnesic patients, such for example as those suffering from Korsakoff syndrome. This is a condition produced by a vitamin deficiency which in turn results from chronic alcoholism. The patient may show grossly defective memory, being unable to orient himself in time or place, and be quite incapable of recognizing for example someone who had just spent several hours working with him. Typically, working memory may be intact, as evidenced by unimpaired recency effects and normal memory span. Ability to learn lists of words however would be grossly defective, as would memory for pictures or events. It has however become increasingly clear in recent years that such patients do show an ability to learn that is relatively intact for certain tasks.

The classic observation of such learning was made many years ago by the Swiss psychiatrist Claparede, who on one occasion secreted a pin in his hand before shaking hands with a Korsakoff patient on his morning round. Next morning, the patient was reluctant to shake hands, but appeared to have no direct recollection of the actual incident.

Subsequent research has shown that a wide range of learning tasks may be relatively intact in such globally amnesic patients. These include the ability to learn motor skills, perceptual learning tasks such as reading mirror writing, classical conditioning, and the solving of a range of both perceptual and reasoning problems (see Baddeley, 1982b, for a review). What do such tasks have in common? There is growing agreement that their primary characteristic is that they allow the patient to demonstrate his learning without needing to be aware of when or where the learning took place, information which is typically not available to the amnesic patient. If for example he is learning a skill, then the performance of that skill does not require him to remember having been taught it. It is as if the information has been laid down in memory, the skill is there, but any recollection of the process of learning is lost. Since we tend to judge memory in terms of remembered episodes, it is tempting to conclude that such patients have no memory. In fact, certain aspects of their memory are quite normal and such patients therefore could be taught certain skills which they would retain quite effectively, despite a tendency to deny ever having encountered such a skill. Schacter and his colleagues have recently explored the implication of such preserved learning capacity for rehabilitation, and have shown that it is possible to teach amnesic patients relatively complex skills such as those involved in using a computer (Glisley, Schacter and Tulving 1986)

## AN OVERVIEW OF THE STRUCTURE OF HUMAN MEMORY

While controversy about the detailed analysis of human memory continues, it can reasonably be divided into three broad subsystems, a set of sensory memories that are grossly related to the perceptual processes, and which feed into a working memory system. This is itself quite complex but can be regarded as containing an attentional system, the central executive, aided by a number of subsidiary systems such as the articulatory loop, concerned with speech processing, and the visuospatial sketch pad, concerned with visual imagery. The working memory system is concerned with the temporary storage of information. As such, it contrasts with the long-term memory system which holds information over much longer periods. Long-term memory in turn can usefully be separated into visual and verbal memory, and into long-term memory, for facts, incidents and events, and procedural learning, the acquisition of mental, and physical skills.

## PROCESSING STATES OF MEMORY

Any memory system, be it a biological system such as the human brain, or an electronic system such as a modern computer, must perform three functions. It must allow information to be fed into the system, the **input** or learning stage; it must be able to maintain information, **storage**; and it must be able to access information when appropriate, the process of **retrieval**. The section that follows will consider each of these in turn, primarily using examples from long-term memory, since this is most relevant to memory therapy. It will become clear however, that although it is relatively easy to make a logical distinction between these three stages, in actual practice they interact, a point that can be most readily illustrated using the analogy that is often drawn between a memory system and a library.

INPUT

Obviously for something to be remembered it must have been learned in the first place. The manner of the learning is however crucially important if subsequent recall is to be efficient. More specifically, new material must be categorized and organized with respect to what is already known, just as any adequate library must have an organized cataloguing and shelving system. A library that merely accumulated books in random piles would be virtually unusable.

Having decided that cataloguing is necessary, what principles should be used? A librarian could for example catalogue all red books together and all yellow books, or could classify books according to their size. However while this might be useful if one were simply looking for something to prop up a wobbly table, it would not be a suitable cataloguing system for finding information on a particular subject. If one wishes to access by subject, then obviously items should be coded by subject. The same thing applies in human memory. We typically wish to access information about the world in terms of its meaning, and hence long-term memory tends to categorize and work most efficiently on the basis of meaning. However, meaning is by no means the only thing that needs to be stored. If we wish to remember someone's name, then obviously we need to store verbal or phonological information as well as semantic and episodic information about that person. The term coding is used to refer to the processing of information during learning, and has formed perhaps the most active area of research in human memory over the last decade. What factors have proved to be important?

## Attention

If the person is to learn something then he or she must attend to it. While this may seem obvious, there are occasional claims to the contrary, as for example in the case of sleep teaching, where it has been claimed that information presented while sleeping is absorbed and retained. Unfortunately, in practice, such short cuts to painless learning simply do not seem to work.

The role of attention in learning is a very central one. If for example a person attempts to split his attention between a learning task and something quite different, such as dealing cards into different suits, then the more difficult the dealing task the less he will remember of the words. A minor exception to this is the recency effect, which seems insensitive to division of attention. At a practical level, this suggests that watching the television with one eye and reading a book with the other might allow you the comforting feeling that you have remembered what you read in the line before, but will nevertheless grossly reduce the amount that you retain subsequently of whatever you read, or watched.

Clearly then, patients who have difficulty in sustaining attention will have difficulty in learning. Hence patients with frontal lobe damage or patients suffering from dementia are likely to show poor learning unless considerable efforts are made to keep their attention on the task in hand.

## Intention to learn

This might appear to be an important variable, but in fact it is not. Experimental studies have shown that provided subjects attend to the material and process it in an appropriate way, it does not matter whether they are trying to learn or not. Similarly trying to learn but performing inappropriate learning strategies will lead to relatively little improvement. What is important is what the patient does and how, but not why he does it.

## Organization

Learning is crucially dependent on organization of material. Just as the core of a good library is its cataloguing system, so the essence of a good memory is the way in which material is organized during learning. People who are expert in a particular area will already have a rich and well-organized cataloguing system which will enable them to acquire new material more easily and more rapidly. Hence an expert chess player can acquire in a single glimpse of a game more information than a novice player can acquire in four or five times as many glimpses. A football enthusiast can hear the results and recall them much more effectively than someone who has a merely passing interest in football, and an electronics expert can 'read' and remember a circuit diagram that would require vastly longer for the amateur to learn. In all these cases, the new material is organized in terms of what already exists, and efficient learning should attempt to take advantage of what is already known in order to graft on new material.

## Levels of processing

As we saw earlier, the immediate recall of lists of words seems to depend heavily on the sound or spoken characteristics of those words, while long-term learning appears to rely more on semantic coding. Craik and Lockhart (1972) generalized this type of finding by suggesting that material can be processed at a range of different 'depths', and that the deeper the processing the better the retention. Suppose I were to present you with a list of words, requiring you to answer questions about each word. For some words I might ask you questions that required only a relatively superficial processing of the word; for example 'Is the word LAMB written in lower case letters or capitals?' Or I might ask a question requiring slightly deeper processing; 'Does the word "dog" rhyme with "log"?' Or I might ask a question that required yet deeper semantic processing: 'Would the word "pig" be a suitable completion for the sentence 'The farmer went to the market to buy a . . .'?

It proves to be the case that the most superficial processing in terms of letter characteristics leads to poorest recall, processing in terms of rhyme somewhat better, while semantic processing leads to the best retention. While the interpretation of this result is still controversial, there is no doubt that as a rule of thumb, deeper encoding does tend to lead to better learning.

What is meant by deeper encoding? This presents a problem, certainly at a theoretical level. However at a practical level the following features appear to characterize efficient deep processing.

1. Elaboration: working on the detail of material and relating it to what one already knows appears to enhance learning.
2. Compatibility: material that is consistent with existing knowledge is easier to learn than inconsistent material, and neutral material can be learnt best by attempting to relate it to what is already known.
3. Self-reference: learners who are asked to judge how material relates to themselves seem to remember it better than if they are required to judge its relevance to other people.

It seems likely that methods such as the PQRST approach that have been shown to facilitate the comprehension and retention of prose in patients with memory problems (Wilson, 1987a, Chapter 9) derive much of their effect from inducing deeper processing.

### Distribution of practice in learning

The principle of a little and often is a good learning precept. This applies at two levels. First, if you are trying to teach over a long period of time, then it is a mistake to try to pack too much into each individual day. A study on learning to type compared training regimes involving one hour a day, two hours a day and four hours a day. Both the learning rate and subsequent retention was best for the one hour a day group and worst for the four-hour group.

A similar principle operates at the micro level. Suppose for example you were trying to teach someone the name of a person. If you present this information twice, then presenting it twice in quick succession leads to less learning than presenting it twice with a few minutes' delay in between. In learning it is important to keep track of what has been learned by including frequent tests, and if you test recall after a short delay, rather than a long one, the patient is more likely to be able to recall it. A successful recall will have two advantages, one a motivational encouragement, and the other due to the fact that the recall itself will function as a second learning trial. Bearing this in mind, the optimal teaching strategy is to begin by presenting and testing after a short delay, but gradually build up the interval as learning proceeds, aiming always to test the item at the longest interval for which the subject is likely to be able to recall it. Such a strategy hence combines early success and encouragement with a gradually increasing distribution of practice. (See Landauer and Bjork, 1978, for a more detailed description of this approach.)

## STORAGE

Once information is registered in memory, then it must be stored until subsequently needed. Forgetting over time may either represent loss of that information or increased difficulty in retrieving it. Reverting to our library analogy, loss of information would presumably represent books either being thrown away, or possibly becoming unreadable due to fading print. The issue of how much forgetting, if any, occurs because of loss rather than inaccessibility remains controversial.

The typical form of a forgetting curve was first demonstrated by the German psychologist Hermann Ebbinghaus as long ago as 1885. The function is exponential, with forgetting rapid at first, becoming more and more gradual as time elapses. In general, rate of forgetting appears to be surprisingly stable across different groups of people. Hence grossly amnesic Korsakoff patients may show very impaired learning, but once something is learnt, subsequently it is remembered just as well as in the case of normals. The same combination of poor learning and normal subsequent retention is also found in patients suffering from closed head injury, and the normal elderly (Baddeley, Harris and

Sunderland, 1987) as well as for Alzheimer's Disease patients (Kopelman, 1985).

It is almost certainly the case that memory registration and storage depends on some form of neurochemical change. There is a growing body of evidence to suggest that patients suffering from dementia exhibit both memory problems and deficits in certain potentially important neurotransmitters (Kopelman, 1986). This has encouraged the search for drugs that might allow the deficit to be made good, so far with relatively limited success (see Chapter 7 for a more detailed discussion).

## RETRIEVAL

Memory systems, like libraries, can only be regarded as successful if they can both store information and retrieve it on request. There is no doubt that some forgetting occurs, not because the information is lost, but merely because it becomes increasingly difficult to retrieve. An everyday example of this is the tip-of-the-tongue effect in which one tries to remember something, often a name, which one is certain one knows but simply cannot produce at the time. One can often be quite successful in saying how many syllables there are in the name and recall some of its letters, and yet not be able to produce the item. When it is presented, one typically has no difficulty in recognizing that it is the correct response.

What determines whether an item can or cannot be retrieved? One factor we have discussed already, namely how it was encoded in the first place. Casual and disorganized encoding tends to lead to unreliable retrieval. However, whatever the manner of encoding, retrieval seems to be best if the encoding situation is reinstated. This aspect of memory has been explored most vigorously by Tulving who has formulated what he terms the *Encoding Specificity Principle* (Tulving 1983).

## Encoding specificity

As mentioned earlier, this states that retrieval will be optimal when it occurs in the same context as learning. This can be illustrated most simply using the case of environmental context.

## Context dependent memory

The philosopher Locke describes the case of a young man who took dancing lessons. The lessons occurred in a room containing an old trunk. The young man learnt to dance quite effectively in that room but 'though in that chamber he could dance excellently well, yet it was only while that trunk was there; nor could he perform well in any other place, unless that or some other such trunk had its due position in the room'. (Locke, 1690; Everyman's Library Edition (1961) Vol. 1, pp. 339–40).

A similar effect of environmental context was observed by a colleague Duncan Godden and me in the case of deep-sea divers (Godden and Baddeley, 1975). We taught our divers a list of words either on land or underwater, and required them to recall the words in either the same environment or the different one. Our divers learnt a similar amount on land or underwater, but recalled about 40% less when they attempted to remember the words in the opposite environment to that in which they learnt them. However, when instead of requiring them to recall the words we used a recognition measure in which they had to pick the previously presented words out of a list, our context-dependency effect disappeared (Godden and Baddeley, 1980). They recognized the same number regardless of whether recognition occurred in the same environment as learning or the opposite. This suggests that the words had indeed been stored, and that accessing them was helped by reinstating the learning context. Under recognition conditions, since the words were presented to the subject, access was not a problem; the difficulty lay in deciding whether the accessed word had been presented earlier in the experiment. The contextual effects we observed with recall were particularly large, presumably because the difference between being on land and underwater is particularly dramatic. There is however considerable evidence to suggest that reliable though less marked effects occur with less pronounced environmental changes.

## State-dependent memory

If instead of changing the external environment within which a person is operating, one changes his internal environment by means of drugs, a similar effect occurs. It has for example been observed that alcoholics who hide money and liquor while drunk, may be unable to remember where it was hidden when sober, but recall when drunk again (Goodwin *et al.*, 1969); what is learned when drunk is apparently best recalled drunk. Again, as with context-dependent memory, when subjects are tested by recognition rather than recall, the effect of state during learning disappears (Eich, 1980).

Similar effects are associated with changes in emotional state; sad memories are easier to recall in a sad mood than when happy, and vice versa (Bower, 1981). Such a process probably makes it hard for depressive patients to escape their depression since their memory for sad events tends to be better than that for happy incidents in their earlier life (Teasdale, 1983).

## Retrieval cues

So far we have talked about the contextual effects in learning provided by the subject's environment, either external or internal. The psychological context in which learning occurs can however have an equally marked effect. An extensive series of studies by Tulving have developed the concept of a *retrieval cue*. Retrieval cues are fragments of the original learning experience which can serve to prompt recall or recognition. They can be used to explore the way in which the original learning took place.

Let us begin with a fairly extreme case. Suppose you are trying to help a patient remember a word so that it can be recalled later on request. Let us begin by supposing that it is a word that has two meanings like *jam* (as in strawberry jam and traffic jam), and that you encourage one of these interpretations during learning. You might for example say 'The next word is "jam", as in: "They had jam for tea."' Somewhat later the patient fails to remember it and you give him a hint. If you give him the hint of 'strawberry' or 'something you might have for tea', this will very probably help him. If on the other hand you give him a hint concerned with the other meaning of jam such as 'traffic', then this is likely to actively reduce the probability that he will remember the word. Indeed, under these circumstances, it is often possible to show him the word and he will deny that it is the one that was presented. What this means is that what he has stored is the meaning of the word not the word itself.

If this effect only occurred when words have two meanings, it would be of theoretical but not great practical importance. However, similar effects occur when different features of a word with only one meaning are stressed. Suppose you had used the word piano, and given as an illustrative sentence 'The strong man lifted the piano'. You would find that 'something heavy' was a very effective hint, but that 'something tuneful' was not. What the subject encodes appears to be those aspects of the stimulus that are highlighted by the context. If the retrieval cue emphasizes some other feature, then it is unlikely to help and may indeed actively hinder.

These results clearly show that patients are likely to be helped by hints, but that these should be carefully chosen, bearing in mind the context in which the material was learned. The principle underlying them however has a much more general and important implication for therapy. The implication is captured by the term 'encoding variability' which is the converse of encoding specificity.

## Encoding variability

A constant problem for therapy of any kind is the question of the extent to which improvements observed in the clinic actually generalize to the patient's everyday life. For example, a study of stroke patients showed that the level of performance on activities of daily living they demonstrated in hospital was substantially greater than the activities they actually accomplished for themselves when they subsequently returned home (Sheikh, Smith and Meade, 1978).

There are of course many possible reasons for this, but one of them is the phenomenon of encoding specificity; all too often, what is learnt in one specific context does not generalize to others. One way of minimizing this danger is to ensure that, once a skill has been acquired, it should be utilized and practised in as wide a range of environments as possible. Ideally of course, these should closely resemble the environment in which the skill will be practised outside the hospital, but if this is not possible, a wide range of hospital contexts is better than confining practice to one situation.

## CONCLUSIONS

Memory theory cannot and will not ever be in a position to provide the therapist with simple recipes for treating memory problems. What theory can do is to provide a broad orientation within which to understand something of the patient's deficit, and suggest possible techniques and strategies for ameliorating these problems. We have in the last decade learnt a good deal about how to enhance learning and memory within the laboratory. To what extent these techniques are applicable in the clinic, and more importantly in the world outside, remains to be seen. There is certainly no guarantee of success; indeed it is by no means certain at this stage whether the retraining of cognitive function in brain-damaged patients will ever be an important and significant component of therapy. It is however certainly a possibility that needs to be explored extensively and evaluated thoroughly and carefully. Such an exploration and evaluation needs the combined skills of both the theorist and the clinician.

## REFERENCES

Atkinson, R.C., and Shiffrin, R.M. (1971) The control of short-term memory. *Scientific American*, **225**, 82–90.

Baddeley, A.D. (1966a) Short-term memory for word sequences as a function of acoustic, semantic and formal similarity. *Quarterly Journal of Experimental Psychology*, **18**, 362–5.

Baddeley, A.D. (1966b) The influence of acoustic and semantic similarity on long-term memory for word sequences. *Quarterly Journal of Experimental Psychology*, **18**, 302–9.

Baddeley, A.D. (1982a) *Your Memory: A User's Guide*. Penguin Books Harmondsworth, Middlesex.

Baddeley, A.D. (1982b) Amnesia: A minimal model and an interpretation. in L. Cermak (ed.), *Human Memory and Amnesia*. Lawrence Erlbaum Associates, Hillsdale, N.J.

Baddeley, A.D. (1982c) Implications of neuropsychological evidence for theories of normal memory. *Philosophical Transactions of the Royal Society London* B, **298**, 59–72.

Baddeley A.D. (1986) *Working Memory* Oxford, OUP.

Baddeley, A.D., Harris, J., Sunderland, A., Watts, K. and Wilson, B. (1987) Closed head injury and memory, in H. Levin (ed.), *Neurobehavioral Recovery from Head Injury.* Oxford University Press, New York. 295–317.

Baddeley, A.D., and Hitch, G.J. (1974) Working memory, in G.A. Bower (ed.), *The Psychology of Learning and Motivation*, **8**, Academic Press, New York.

Baddeley, A.D., Logie, R., Bressi, S., Della Sala, S. and Spinnler, H. (1986) Dementia and working memory, *Quarterly Journal of Experimental Psychology*, **38A**, 603–18.

Baddeley, A.D., Papagno, C. and Vallar, G. (1988) When long-term learning depends on short-term storage. *Journal of Memory and Language*, **27**, 586–95.

Baddeley, A.D., Vallar, G. and Wilson, B.A. (1987) Sentence comprehension and phonological memory: Some neuropsychological evidence, in M. Coltheart (ed.), *Attention and Performance XII: The Psychology of Reading.* Lawrence Erlbaum Associates, London. 509–29.

Baddeley, A.D., and Warrington, E.K. (1970) Amnesia and the distinction between long- and short-term memory. *Journal of Verbal Learning and Verbal Behavior*, **9**, 176–89.

Bower, G.H. (1981) Mood and memory. *American Psychologist*, **36**, 129–48.

Craik, F.I.M., and Lockhart, R.S. (1972) Levels of processing: a framework for memory research. *Journal of Verbal Learning and Verbal Behavior*, **11**, 671–84.

Craik, F.I.M., and Watkins, M.J. (1973) The role of rehearsal in short-term memory. *Journal of Verbal Learning and Verbal Behavior*, **12**, 599–607.

Eich, J.E. (1980) The cue-dependent nature of state-dependent retrieval. *Memory and Cognition*, **8**, 157–73.

Farah M.J. (1988) Is visual imagery really visual? Overlooked evidence from neuropsychology. *Psychological Review*, **95**, 307–17.

Glisky E, Schacter, D. and Tulving, E. (1986) Computer learning by memory impaired patients: acquisition and retention of complex knowledge. *Neuropsychologia*, **24**, 313–28.

Godden, D., and Baddeley, A.D. (1975) Context-dependent memory in two natural environments: on land and under water. *British Journal of Psychology*, **66**, 325–31.

Godden, D., and Baddeley, A.D. (1980) When does context influence recognition memory? *British Journal of Psychology*, **71**, 99–104.

Goodwin, D.W., Powell, B., Bremer, D., Hoine, H., and Stern, J. (1969) Alcohol and recall: state dependent effects in man. *Science*, **163**, 1358.

Hersen, M., and Barlow, D.H. (1976) *Single Case Experimental Designs:*

*Strategies for Studying Behavior Change*. Elmsford, Pergamon, New York.

Jones, M.K. (1974) Imagery as a mnemonic aid after left temporal lobectomy: contrast between material-specific and generalized memory disorders. *Neuropsychologia*, 12, 21–30.

Kopelman, M.D. (1985) Rates of forgetting in Alzheimer-type dementia and Korsakoff's syndrome. *Neuropsychologia*, 3, 623–38.

Kopelman, M.D. (1986) The cholinergic neurotransmitter system in human memory and dementia: A review. *Quarterly Journal of Experimental Psychology*, 38A, 535–74.

Landauer, T.K., and Bjork, R.A. (1978) Optimum rehearsal patterns and name learning, in M.M. Gruneberg, P.E. Morris and R.N. Sykes (eds.), *Practical Aspects of Memory*. Academic Press, London.

Locke, J. (1690) *Everyman's Library Edition* (1961) 1, 339–40.

Peterson, L.R., and Peterson, M.J. (1959) Short-term retention of individual verbal items. *Journal of Experimental Psychology*, 58, 193–8.

Postman, L., and Phillips, L.W. (1965) Short-term temporal changes in free recall. *Quarterly Journal of Experimental Psychology*, 17, 132–8.

Rabbitt, P. (1981) Cognitive psychology needs models for changes in performance with old age, in J.B. Long and A.D. Baddeley (eds.), *Attention and Performance IX*. Erlbaum and Hillsdale, N.J.

Shallice, T. (1979) Neuropsychological research and the fractionation of memory systems, in L. Nilsson (ed.), *Perspectives in Memory Research*. L. Erlbaum, Hillsdale, N.J.

Shallice, T., and Warrington, E.K. (1970) Independent functioning of verbal memory stores: a neuropsychological study. *Quarterly Journal of Experimental Psychology*, 22, 261–73.

Sheikh, K., Smith, D.S., Meade, T.W., and Brennan, P.J. (1978) Methods and problems of a stroke rehabilitation trial. *British Journal of Occupational Therapy*, 41, 262–5.

Teasdale, J.D. (1983) Affect and accessibility. *Philosophical Transactions of the Royal Society of London B*, 302, 403–12.

Tulving E (1983) *Elements of Episodic Memory*. Oxford, OUP.

Vallar, G., and Baddeley, A.D. (1984) Fractionation of working memory. Neuropsychological evidence for a phonological short-term store. *Journal of Verbal Learning and Verbal Behavior*. 23 151–61.

Welford, A.T. (1980) Memory and age: a perspective view, in L.W. Poon, J.L. Fozard, L.S. Cermak, D. Arenberg, and L.W. Thompson (eds.), *New Directions in Memory and Aging*. Erlbaum, Hillsdale, N.J. pp. 1–17.

Wilson, B. (1982) Success and failure in memory training following a cerebral vascular accident. *Cortex*, 18, 581–94.

Wilson B.A. and Baddeley A.D. (1988) Semantic episodic and autobiographical memory in a post meningitic amnesic patient. *Brain and Cognition* 8 31–46.

Wilson, B.A. (1987a) *Rehabilitation of Memory*. Guilford Press, New York.

Wilson, B.A. (1987b) Single case experimental designs in neuro-psychological rehabilitation. *Journal of Clinical and Experimental Neuropsychology*, **9**, 527–44.

## Chapter 2

# Assessment for rehabilitation

### NADINA B. LINCOLN and NEIL BROOKS

The role of assessment in rehabilitation varies from department to department. In some cases patients are given a series of structured tasks and on the basis of performance on these tasks a rehabilitation programme is planned and its effectiveness is monitored by repetition of the assessment tasks. In others, the assessment and treatment stages cannot be clearly differentiated and abilities are assessed and treated on the basis of observations made throughout the rehabilitation programme. In the latter case monitoring the effectiveness of treatment is usually based on observation of whether the patient appears to have improved on the activities.

If we are going to separate assessment techniques from intervention strategies then we need first to consider what is meant by assessment. In this chapter, assessment is considered as a structured programme of observations made by the rehabilitation team. These observations may be used to identify the difficulties that a person has, to measure their severity, determine the impact they have on daily life and to monitor any changes in ability that occur, either as a result of spontaneous recovery or in response to treatment. In order to decide which assessment techniques to use we need to consider four basic questions. We need to consider why assessments are being carried out, who is going to do them, when they are going to do them and what functions need to be assessed. The answers to these questions will determine the techniques that are to be used on any given occasion.

## WHY ARE ASSESSMENTS CARRIED OUT?

It is all too easy to carry out an assessment simply because it is the one carried out in the department. Such assessments may be carried out merely to justify the existence of the department: this is not adequate, but is distressingly common nevertheless. If greater consideration is given to why the assessment is being carried out, then this unnecessary routine can be avoided.

One of the main reasons for assessing a patient, particularly in the early stages, is to identify what his or her abilities and deficits are. Such an assessment will include a wide range of practical skills and, when considering patients with memory problems, a wide range of cognitive abilities. These assessments tend to be carried out using standardized procedures, for which there is some indication of how a person of any given age, intelligence level or social background would be likely to perform. These include standardized tests, rating scales and questionnaires. The information gathered can be used to plan the rehabilitation programme because it indicates which skills a person is likely to have lost. Repetition of these procedures will indicate the extent to which the patient has improved either as a result of treatment, spontaneous recovery or increased familiarity with the test materials or test regime.

The second purpose of assessments may be to identify functions hypothesized to underlie observed deficits. This is an important point, as the reasons for failure on a test may be many. The patient who, for example, cannot complete a task in rehabilitation may have a number of deficits ranging from general slowness, to an attentional or concentration deficit, to low drive and motivation, to poor arousal. A knowledge of the underlying deficits will enable rehabilitation staff to plan a treatment programme tailored uniquely to that patient rather than the broad range of patients who come through the department.

Although the purpose may be to identify and assess cognitive deficits after brain damage, much of the research work has been of an atheoretical and rather *ad hoc* nature; the measures used are often related only peripherally, if at all, to current cognitive theorizing, and this inevitably means that it is very difficult to specify exactly why a given patient has a given cognitive deficit. There are exceptions to this general rule, for example, the use of a short- and long-term memory model (Brooks, 1975; Parker and Serrats, 1976; Wilson, Brooks and Phillips, 1982). Other exceptions would include the excellent work of Van Zomeren and his colleagues on attention deficits (Van Zomeren, Brouwer and Deelman, 1983), and Levin's use of a hemispheric disconnection model in assessing deficits after head injury (Levin, Grossman, Sarwar and Meyers, 1981). With these exceptions, however, clinical assessment of cognitive functions, particularly after head injury, has proceeded almost entirely independently of current theoretical views about cognition. The assessment of more focal lesions has not been atheoretical to the same extent, as the excellent work carried out by Warrington and her colleagues (Warrington, 1971; Warrington, 1974; Warrington and James, 1967) illustrates.

While *ad hoc* clinical tests will undoubtedly identify major deficits, the tests are often too multifactorial to allow any informed judgement about precisely why a patient fails on the test. A 'frontal' patient and one with a left temporal lesion may both fail the same verbal learning test, with apparently identical severities of deficit. The underlying reasons for failure, however, may be very varied indeed, demanding entirely different procedures for their further elucidation, and different approaches to rehabilitation and management.

The third reason for assessing a patient is to identify the effect any deficits observed have on his everyday life. The skills required in the outside world are very different from those required in a hospital. Some patients may cope much better in the familiar surroundings of their own homes than in the occupational therapy department, surrounded by other people with an unfamiliar arrangement of household equipment. In other cases, patients may be able to carry out routine daily activities in the company of others simply because they get necessary clues from what others are doing. However, on their own at home such clues may not be available and the person may be unable to cope with simple routine self-care activities. Alternatively, the patient may fail to cope because the carer at home may prefer to do things

for the patient rather than waiting for the completion of
a slow and inaccurate performance. Andrews and Stewart
(1979) investigated this in a series of stroke patients, and
found that performance in activities of daily living in the
clinic was better than in the patient's own home. Indeed,
whereas there were a number of ADL areas in which
the patient performed better in the clinic than at home,
the reverse was not observed. It is therefore necessary to
assess people's performance in the environment in which
their skills will be needed as well as in the rehabilitation
department. This applies to many social skills as well as
simple daily activities. Can the person cope with a noisy
office, a crowded works canteen, climbing three flights
of stairs to his flat when the lifts are not working, and
asking for a pint of beer in a pub with an unfamiliar
landlord?

Discrepancies between performance on standard tasks in
a hospital setting and performance in the outside world
have recently received considerable attention. Sunderland,
Harris and Baddeley (1983) carried out a study to investigate whether laboratory tests predict everyday memory.
They took three groups of patients. Two of the groups
consisted of patients who had received severe head injury
(assessed within a few months of injury in one group and
between two and eight years after injury in the other).
The third group consisted of accident victims who had
suffered recent orthopaedic injuries, but claimed never to
have been knocked unconscious. The three groups were
similar in terms of type of accident, socio-economic status and age. All patients were tested on an objective test
battery and were asked to complete a questionnaire to
assess the incidence of memory failures. In addition, a
relative or close friend of each patient was interviewed
and asked to estimate the frequency of memory failures
using the same questionnaire items. Both the patient and
the relative were given a check-list at the end of the interview to complete on seven consecutive days following the
interview indicating whether that form of memory failure had happened to the patient each day. Performance
on the objective tests correlated significantly with scores
on the relatives' questionnaire for the non-head injured

and the long-term head injured group, but not for the recently head injured subjects who had yet to reach a stable state. The authors report that correlations between test performance and questionnaire were higher for tests involving prose recall and paired associate learning than for tests of visual memory, and they suggest that the lower correlations with visual memory tests may have been due to the low salience of visual errors in everyday life. In addition, the patients' questionnaires showed the least agreement with the checklists and the objective tests illustrating the problem of validity of self-report with these patients. Further evidence comes from Brooks (1979) who used a simpler version of the Sunderland questionnaire, and found no association between clinical memory test performance and questionnaire score, at three months after injury, but significant correlations between questionnaire and both verbal and non-verbal memory measures at six months after injury.

The fourth reason for assessment is to identify the goals of the rehabilitation programme. It is not enough merely to assess the patient in the laboratory or clinic, to identify the nature of the deficit and the effects it has on everyday life, and to monitor progress. It is also necessary to identify which skills need to be acquired and in what order. Some deficits may be relatively trivial in terms of their impact on actual abilities, yet put considerable emotional strain on the relatives of the patient. It may be necessary to treat these before the more obvious practical deficits. For example, a patient who repeatedly asks the same question or tells the same story may impose far more emotional strain on relatives due to this reiteration rather than to his inability to carry out activities unsupervised. Priorities need to be established both from the patients' and the relatives' points of view when deciding the over all treatment plan. Social circumstances may change during rehabilitation so that the goals identified at the beginning may become secondary to others which have subsequently assumed importance. So, not only do the initial goals need to be specified, but they also need to be reviewed from time to time to check that they are still appropriate.

## WHO MAKES ASSESSMENTS?

Initially assessments are made by the team most closely involved with the patient's rehabilitation. This will include the physicians, surgeons, nurses, rehabilitation therapists, psychologists and social workers. Each member of the team will consider specific aspects of the patient's abilities which would not necessarily be considered by other members of the team, although in a good, well-integrated team, overlap will (and should) occur. So, for example, the psychologist may be concerned with assessing the nature of the memory deficit (whether the problems are predominantly verbal or visual), the strategy used by the patient to solve a particular task, and the duration of retention of information. The rehabilitation therapists are likely to be more directly concerned with the impact of the memory deficit on the person's life. The occupational therapist may assess whether memory problems affect the patient's ability to carry out routine domestic chores. For example Mrs AW had difficulty following a recipe because, between reading the instructions in the recipe book and going to pick up the item from the shelf, she forgot what she was supposed to be doing next. The speech therapist may assess the effect of a deficit on communication skills, for example, the problems encountered by the patient who is unable to understand a short passage in the newspaper because he forgets earlier information as he reads through the paper. The physiotherapist may find the patient is unable to practise a series of exercises on his own because, even though the exercises have been demonstrated many times before, the sequence is either too long or too complex for the patient to recall more than the first few stages. Nurses may observe that the patient has problems with following through a sequence of activities such as getting up, washing, dressing and going to breakfast, because he loses track of what he has done, and what has yet to be done.

The role of the family as suppliers of information should not be neglected, and family members can fill in simple ratings and check lists about behaviours outside the rehabilitation setting. This is important because some things never or rarely happen in a hospital setting, yet observation of how the patient copes with unusual problems at home may provide valuable insight into the nature of the difficulties. Unexpected callers at the house, a changed appointment time or a diversion on a shopping route because of a burst water-main may disrupt a person's routine to the extent that difficulties which had hitherto been unnoticed become very apparent. Similarly, if the patient had been employed at the time of the injury, then information from the employer may be particularly valuable, not only in giving further information about the patient's strengths and weaknesses in employment-related areas, but also, as rehabilitation progresses, in assessing the patient's acquisition of the skills necessary for return to work.

It is important to note that there may be great discrepancies in the information supplied by different people, and the likely sources of these discrepancies need to be identified. One possibility is that a discrepancy is due simply to an unreliable rating scale, and this is unfortunately a very common feature of scales used in rehabilitation departments, in which the questions are often ambiguous and open to widely divergent interpretation by different members of the team. Furthermore, if the patient and relative are both used as direct sources of information about the patient's functioning, discrepancies may be particularly large in areas representing behavioural and psychological functions (McKinlay and Brooks, 1984). However, in some instances there may also be quite marked discrepancies in patients' reported physical abilities in activities of daily living and those of relatives (Lincoln, 1981). Such discrepancies as these not only highlight areas of particular concern for different people in contact with the patient but they may also indicate the extent to which the patient is aware of his own difficulties.

WHEN SHOULD ASSESSMENTS BE CARRIED OUT?

Assessments should be made initially as near as possible to the beginning of the rehabilitation process. This allows for an assessment of the effectiveness of rehabilitation, or of spontaneous recovery, but the earlier the assessment is made then the more difficult it is to make very specific predictions about the patient's likely progress. Very early after a lesion only gross and short-term predictions can be made, but as time progresses the accuracy and uniqueness of the prediction increases as the patient comes nearer to his final level. However, as the patient nears this level the less change is likely and the less useful the assessment. There is no easy answer here.

The timing of the assessment is to some extent determined by the purpose of the assessment. In the early stages one is more likely to be concerned with identifying abilities and deficits and functions assumed to be underlying the deficits. The recovery of these will then be monitored. As time progresses this type of assessment becomes less important and greater emphasis is placed on the effect the deficits have on daily life. Later still, assessments will be more specifically directed towards planning the future, such as deciding whether a patient has the skills necessary to return to his former employment or whether some alternative form of employment is appropriate.

The frequency of assessment depends on the function being assessed and the time after the lesion. The earlier the assessments are begun, the more rapid is change likely to be in all areas of functioning. However, some functions do change at different rates from others and this must be taken into account in timing assessments. Gross motor functions and the gross aspects of language may recover quickly to an adequate, though incomplete, level in many patients. This is not the case with memory functions which typically improve more slowly and to a less adequate level (Brooks, 1983; Brooks and Aughton, 1979).

The frequency of reassessment also depends on the type of measure being used. Clearly when familiarity or practice effects are likely to affect performance then the assessment cannot be repeated very often. In contrast, if behavioural observation is being used, the actual assessment procedure is unlikely to affect the patient's performance and so can be repeated as often as desired. Different assessments will be repeated at different stages. It is fairly typical for standardized psychological tests to be carried out at one, three, six and twelve months post-injury, activities of daily living to be assessed at four- or six-weekly intervals and observational rating scales to be carried out daily.

WHAT FUNCTIONS NEED TO BE ASSESSED?

The aim of this section is to describe some of the functions which need to be assessed (for a more comprehensive list see Wilson (in press),) and also to illustrate some of the techniques which are currently available. At a very general level, the assessment should encompass the full range of functions known to be important in achieving competent activities of daily living and adequate interpersonal cognitive or vocational performance in the outside world. Many functions likely to be important can be specified from clinical experience or simply from common sense. For example, memory, perceptual deficits, language, speed of performance, dexterity, motor power and sensory loss can all be seen to have direct implications for adequate performance in the outside world.

This list can be supplemented by those which are known directly to contribute to vocational failure. These have been studied in some detail by Lewinsohn and Graf (1973) who found that failure of occupational placement after various kinds of disability was predicted by disturbances in locomotion, social immaturity, inadequacy, lack of emotional support at home, suspicion, poor motivation, poor attention span, depression and unrealistic goals. Interestingly, in addition to these deficits, there were a number of problems or items which occurred frequently in patients with brain damage, but were *not* found to be significant in predicting vocational success, or predicted only weakly. These were deficits in speech, reading and writing and also rigidity, anxiety, being easily upset, being too slow and having motor incoordination. On factor analysis, various factors were found to be predictive of vocational outcome. Behaviour disorders and cognitive difficulties accounted for the largest proportion of the variability. Other factors accounting for slightly less of the variability in outcome were environmental problems, motor control, age, neuroticism and personal appearance. A number of these areas are easy to assess in the clinic. For example, some may be measured by means of standardized questionnaires (neuroticism), behavioural observation (personal appearance), careful history (environmental problems, age) and physical examination (motor control). The remaining areas, cognitive disturbance and behaviour disorders, which together account for the largest proportions of variance, are less easy to assess, but worth considering in more detail. The emphasis will be placed on the assessment of memory problems since this is the central focus of this book. However, it must be borne in mind that memory problems should always be assessed in conjunction with other cognitive deficits and many of the limitations of the techniques used apply equally to other areas of cognitive disturbance.

### Practical assessment of memory functions

The problem of assessing any cognitive function is to know the areas which can safely be left out. Brain damage of different aetiologies, different velocities, different sites and occurring at different ages can have markedly different effects on cognitive functions. Memory and learning are two functions which are most commonly affected and therefore it is likely that any neuropsychological assessment for rehabilitation will incorporate some assessment of these functions. In addition, their effect on daily life, employment and interpersonal relationships must be considered.

The first stage of memory assessment is to identify which aspects of memory are affected and which are relatively intact. This is usually done using psychological tests or at least tests developed by psychologists. There is a myth that only psychologists may use many of the standard test procedures. While it does hold some truth in relation to restricted circulation tests such as the Wechsler Adult Intelligence Scales (WAIS, WAIS-R) (Wechsler, 1955, 1981), many of the psychological tests used in clinical practice could be administered by other members of the rehabilitation team provided they have the necessary training to enable them to interpret the results obtained. In a review of memory testing, Mayes (1986) points out that memory disorders are heterogeneous and the assessment procedure should reflect this. Tests should be selected which indicate both the severity of the disorder and the kind of memory which is impaired.

Memory has to be evaluated in relation to a patient's general level of intellectual functioning, particularly his premorbid level. In most cases assessment of IQ does not contribute anything materially to the information gained from assessing individual cognitive functions. However, it does provide a baseline against which other functions may be compared. Tests used for this purpose include the WAIS-R (Weschler, 1981), Progressive Matrices and Mill Hill Vocabulary (Raven, 1958). Another which may help provide an indication of premorbid intellectual level is a measure of reading ability, the National Adult Reading Test (Nelson, 1982).

Once the likely premorbid intelligence level has been established it is possible to consider whether different aspects of memory functioning are impaired relative to this level. The ideal would be to have a battery of memory tests tapping different aspects of memory functioning. Although some batteries are available, none is entirely satisfactory and for this reason many clinicians use a selection of different tests. The selection of measures is largely a matter of personal preference but some of the more commonly used procedures will be described.

The most widely used battery of memory tests is the Wechsler Memory Scale (WMS) (Wechsler, 1945). This consists of seven subtests: Personal and Current Information, Orientation, Mental Control, Logical Memory, Memory Span, Visual Reproduction and Associate Learning. These together provide a summary score of memory functioning, the memory quotient. Despite many criticisms about its validity (for reviews see Erickson and Scott, 1977; Prigatano, 1978; Loring and Papanicolaou, 1987) it provides a relatively short screening assessment which can be used to detect memory impairment in many patients (Brooks, 1976). In its original form it was least sensitive to impairments of memory for visual material, but the WMS has been revised (Wechsler, 1987) and includes new subtests designed specifically to assess visual memory. The WMS-R also includes delayed recall of both visual and verbal material as part of the standard administration. Scores from the WMS-R are combined to five indices: general memory index, attention/concentration index, visual memory index, verbal memory index and delayed recall index. The revised WMS is appropriate for clients between 16 and 74 years. Another battery of memory tests is the Williams Scale for the Measurement of Memory (Williams, 1968). This includes tests of immediate recall, non-verbal learning (Rey-Davis test), verbal learning (a modified version of Walton and Black's 1957 test), delayed recall and memory for past personal events. This is also open to criticisms about its reliability and validity and has not gained popularity as a clinical tool.

The alternative approach to using a memory battery is to select a range of different tests to measure particular aspects of memory functioning. This has the advantage that the 'best' tests can be used to assess particular memory functions, but because of differences in method of construction and normative samples comparisons between tests often cannot be made. Some of the most commonly used tests are shown in Table 2.1. It can be seen that some of these tests are also included in the memory batteries mentioned above. These are used as individual tests and not necessarily given as part of the full test battery.

The first criterion used in selecting a range of memory tests is whether memory for verbal or non-verbal visual material is being assessed. Although, following cerebral trauma, clearly lateralized cognitive dysfunctions are less common than with stroke, some relative strengths and weaknesses may be observed which assist in the selection of treatment strategy (Chapter 5). The second aspect to be considered in selecting tests is the time interval between the presentation of material and recall. Most examiners include measures of short-term memory, in which recall is directly after the material has been presented and a delayed recall in which material has to be recalled after a delay of ten minutes or more.

The most widely used assessment of verbal memory is the Logical Recall Subtest of the Wechsler Memory Scale (Wechsler, 1945, 1987). Two stories are read to the patient, and then recalled immediately afterwards. In the revised WMS, recall is retested after a half-hour delay. Normative data are available for different age groups of subjects,

**Table 2.1** Table of memory tests used in clinical practice

| Recall | Nature of Material | |
|--------|--------------------|--------------------|
|        | Verbal | Visual |
| Immediate | Digit span | WMS-R visual memory span |
| Short-term | WMS-R logical memory I<br>Recognition memory test words<br>WMS-R verbal paired associates I | Benton visual retention<br>Recognition memory test faces<br>WMS-R figural memory<br><br>WMS-R visual reproduction I<br>WMS-R visual paired associates I<br>Rey-Davis test |
| Delayed | WMS-R logical memory II<br><br>WMS-R verbal paired associates II<br>Williams delayed recall | WMS-R visual reproduction II<br>WMS-R visual paired associates II<br>Rey Osterreith Figure Recall<br>Williams Delayed Recall |

although the data are rather limited. This test has the advantage of high 'face validity', in that its purpose is fairly obvious to the patient who does not feel he is being asked to carry out an obscure or inappropriate task. It also seems to be relatively highly correlated with performance in everyday life (Brooks, 1979; Sunderland *et al.*, 1983; Lincoln and Tinson, 1989). Although the original version of the test did not incorporate the delayed recall of the stories, introduction of this makes the test more sensitive to minor problems in verbal memory and has been shown to be sensitive to the deficits in head-injured patients (Brooks, 1972, 1976, 1983; Brooks *et al.*, 1980).

There are various forms of paired-associate learning tasks which are used to measure verbal learning ability. One of these is derived from the Wechsler battery (1945, 1987) but there are others which vary in terms of the number of word pairs and the degree of association between words in the pairs (Inglis, 1957; Walton and Black, 1957; Brooks and Baddeley, 1976). In all these tasks pairs of words are read to the patient and then one word of the pair is given and the patient asked to recall the word which went with it. The tests differ in the number of times the task is repeated and the scoring method.

Both paired associate tasks and the Wechsler Logical Memory require intelligible speech from the patient. One which does not have this requirement is the words section of the Recognition Memory test (Warrington, 1984). Words are shown to the patient one at a time on cards. The patient is then presented with a list of pairs of words, one word of each pair being from the series shown to the patient. The task of the patient is to select which word of each pair he has just seen. This test is relatively quick and easy to give and also has high face validity. The limitations of this and the Faces section of the Recognition Memory Test are described by Kapur (1987). He considers the test's technical merits and concludes that it has significant deficits in the initial validation studies, ceiling effects and no reliability data. These limit the test for use in routine neuropsychological assessment. However, despite these criticisms, it is becoming widely used in clinical practice and since better alternatives are not available will probably continue to be used.

Delayed recall of verbal material is usually assessed on the Logical Memory test, but an alternative is to use the delayed recall test from the Williams battery. A card with nine pictures is shown to the patient, who is asked to name each picture. After a ten minute delay the patient is asked to recall the pictures, and for those items which he fails he is then given cues. If the patient fails to recall all the pictures after the cues he is then shown a card with 15 pictures and asked to select from these which ones were on the original card. It is not clear to what extent the test measures visual or verbal recall, since the patient both looks at the pictures and names them. However, the test does provide a measure of delayed recall suitable for patients with poor speech, which makes the delayed Logical Memory difficult, or with poor manual dexterity, which makes drawing tasks difficult.

Visual memory tests usually involve the patient drawing geometric shapes from memory, either immediately after having been shown the design or after a delay. The Wechsler Memory Scale includes the Visual Reproduction Subtest for this purpose but it is relatively insensitive to milder problems. A more complex version of this task is the Benton Visual Retention test (Benton, 1974). This consists of a series of ten designs of increasing complexity which are shown to the patient one at a time; the patient is required to reproduce each from memory. There is also a forced choice version of the test which removes the need for adequate manual dexterity to draw (Benton, 1950), but the normative data for this version are rather limited. The revised WMS (Wechsler, 1987) includes three entirely new subtests for visual memory: figural memory, visual paired associates and visual memory span.

Another assessment of non-verbal memory which does not require the patient to draw is the Faces section of the Recognition Memory test (Warrington, 1984). This task is similar to the Words test described earlier, but instead of words the material consists of photographs of people's faces. A less widely used task is the continuous recognition task devised by Kimura (1963). Subjects are shown a series of abstract patterns. They are then shown a longer series which includes some of the original designs which recur in the series. The subject's task is to say which pattern he or she has seen before.

In order to assess memory in physically disabled patients with visual and communication difficulties Lincoln and Staples (1987) developed a maze learning test. Although some normative data are available, the practical usefulness of this test has not been well established.

Procedures for assessing delayed recall of visual material are few. The Williams delayed recall has already been mentioned and there is a delayed recall version of the Benton Visual Retention test (Benton, 1974). Delayed recall of the visual reproduction subtest has been incorporated in the revised WMS (Wechsler, 1987). One other procedure is delayed recall of the Rey-Osterreith figure (Rey, 1959). In this task the patient first has to copy a complex pattern; after a delay, usually a half-hour, he is required to draw the pattern again from memory. Normative data for both this task and the other delayed visual recall tasks are very limited, and again it has the problem that sufficient manual dexterity is required for the patient to be able to draw.

Most tests considered assess anterograde amnesia. Retrograde amnesia is rarely considered. This is probably because, as Parkin (1987) indicates, this is methodologically very difficult to do. He describes the Boston Remote Memory Battery (Albert *et al*, 1979) but this is not suitable for a British population. However, a simple standardized test has been developed (Wilson and Cockburn, 1988) which assesses retrograde amnesia by asking subjects to estimate the prices of common commodities, such as a pint of milk and a first class stamp. It is assumed that the subject answers the questions by referring to the most recent time period available in memory. A more recent test for assessing one aspect of retrograde amnesia namely autobiographical memory appeared in 1990 (Kopelman, Wilson and Baddeley, 1990).

The advantage of these memory tasks is that there are some normative data available, though rarely as much as would be considered ideal. They have also been found to be sensitive to deficits in memory. However, they do not relate closely to some of the difficulties exhibited by patients in daily life. An alternative is to devise tasks which measure the specific deficit of clinical concern. For example, recalling people's names is frequently reported to be difficult. One could obtain photographs of ten faces and tell the patient the name of each person depicted, for example, this is Ann Jones and this is Peter Black, etc. Indeed this precise procedure has been used to assess recovery after head injury in children (Chadwick, Rutter and Schaffer 1981) and it proved to be a very sensitive indicator of impairment. Recall could be tested immediately after presentation and after a delay. Retesting on such a task might be carried out after a few weeks to assess the effect of spontaneous recovery, or after a specific training programme to teach the patient strategies for the recall of people's names. It should be stressed that interpretation of results of such tests requires considerable caution. An improvement in test score does not necessarily mean that recovery of the underlying ability has occurred, as there may be an effect of practice to be accounted for. However, if prior to a treatment programme a patient scored 0 or 1 out of 10 on the test on four consecutive trials at daily intervals and after a training programme that patients scored more than 6 out of 10 on each of four trials, it would be reasonable to consider that the change in score might be related to the effect of the treatment programme. Similar procedures may be devised for learning a route between A and B; recalling a newspaper article; or recalling where in the kitchen items of cutlery and crockery should be put away after washing up. The advantage of this type of procedure is that tasks can be designed to assess the precise problems of an individual patient rather than those found in general in many individuals. Provided that adequate single case experimental designs are used they may also be incorporated into the evaluation of specific treatment techniques (Gianutsos and Gianutsos, 1979; Glasgow, Zeiss and Barrera, 1977; Wilson, 1982) and can then be very powerful research tools.

Some of these practical memory tasks have been incorporated into a standardized test, the Rivermead Behavioural Memory Test (Wilson, Cockburn and Baddeley, 1985). This test was developed to detect impairment of everyday memory functioning and attempts to bridge the gap between laboratory-based measures of memory and assessments obtained by observation and questionnaire. It consists of 11 subtests: remembering a name, remembering a belonging, remembering an appointment, picture recognition, story recall, face recognition, route recall, delivering a message, orientation and date. Each item is scored on a pass or fail basis and a profile score is also recorded to identify how well or badly patients perform on individual parts of the test. The test is easy and quick to administer. It has been found that the RBMT correlates mildly with the WAIS, but strongly with parts of the Wechsler Memory Scale and Recognition Memory Test. Reliability over time and between assessors is good and parallel forms are available. It has been used with various patient groups, including stroke patients (Tinson and Lincoln, 1987), dementia patients (Poon, personal communication) and others (Wilson, 1988).

In order to assess the effect of memory problems in daily life, rating scales, questionnaires and behavioural observations must all be considered. Some published questionnaires are already available, for example, the Subjective Memory Questionnaire (Bennett-Levy and Powell, 1980) and the Inventory of Memory Experiences (Herrman and Neisser, 1978). The questionnaire by Sunderland *et al.* (1983) consists of 35 different types of everyday error. Items were included if they tapped the types of errors that subjects had an opportunity to make in their daily lives. They included cognitive difficulties which pilot work had suggested were prevalent after head injury and included as wide a range of memory failures as possible. The 35 examples were rated for frequency of occurrence 'over the past few weeks', and answers were classified on a five-point scale ranging from 'on every occasion' to 'never'. However, as previously pointed out, inaccuracies of self-report may occur and it is always useful to include observational assessments by other people as well as self-report by the patient. Tasks may be devised to measure more specific aspects of memory function with individual patients. One way of deciding what to assess in detail is to ask the patient to keep a diary for a week of all the occasions when he was aware of forgetting things or when other people point out that he had forgotten something. An example of such a diary is shown in Table 2.2. This shows up problem areas that can be assessed in more detail. Sometimes this may simply involve systematic recording of what a person does. For example, a patient would turn up at the wrong department at the wrong time for treatment sessions, usually because he forgot to look at his programme card or got distracted en route and went to a different place from where he intended to go. Recording of each time he arrived in a treatment room, and whether it was the correct place to be, provided a baseline assessment of the number of times he went to the wrong place and the number of minutes he was late in arriving at the correct place.

Behavioural observations and ratings are useful for identifying problems and evaluating progress with treatment. They may not enable one to predict, with any accuracy greater than that derived from common sense, the likely outcome of rehabilitation or the time course over which improvement may be expected to continue. Attempts have been made to use some of the standardized tests for this purpose, but even then predictions tend to be of broad categories of independence and not specific enough to make concrete recommendations for clinical management of individual patients. These predictive indices are also limited by how little we know about the extent to which rehabilitation actually influences outcome. At present we

**Table 2.2** Diary of a patient with memory problems

| 20 April | | List of Items Forgotten 20 April–22 April |
|---|---|---|
| 12.30 p.m. | 6 | Realized I hadn't put the washing out before leaving home. |
| 1.15 p.m. | 7 | Had to check up washing symbols. |
| 3.30 p.m. | 8 | Remembered that I should have ordered bread for Friday. |
| 4.10 p.m. | 9 | The Asda list was missing from its usual place. |
| 4.35 p.m. | 10 | Rang to order bread but couldn't remember 'wholemeal'. |
| 5.50 p.m. | 11 | Remembered that I should have collected items to be dry cleaned from my sister's. |
| 5.10 p.m. | 12 | Realized tomorrow is our wedding anniversary only when received card from sister. |
| 5.25 p.m. | 13 | Found I hadn't put the oven on earlier as I'd intended to do. |
| 7.35 p.m. | 14 | When helping husband to fill in a form, couldn't remember car number, whereabouts of passport and NAS card. |
| 8.30 p.m. | 15 | Realized I'd forgotten to take Bakewell tart to Mum and Dad's. |
| 11.30 p.m. | 16 | Had to get out of bed to check I'd locked the front door and put the milk bottles out. Remembered I hadn't yet cancelled cream order. |

are not really in a position to predict the extent to which memory deficits will respond to treatment or the restrictions that memory deficits are likely to impose on daily life in even the short-term future. One unfortunate exception to this is the amnesic syndrome which inevitably imposes major and often complete limitations on daily life.

## Assessment of related functions

Memory assessment cannot be considered in isolation and many other cognitive functions will affect performance on memory tasks and the ability of a patient to cope with memory deficits in daily life.

Perceptual functions are more often assessed in stroke patients than in head-injured patients, but even in the latter group, deficits quite often occur, particularly early after injury. If a person's perceptual abilities are impaired then this is likely to affect memory for visual material and ability to use visually based strategies to cope with memory problems. Various techniques are available for assessing perceptual problems, such as copying the Rey-Osterreith complex figure (Rey, 1959), Unusual Views (Warrington and Taylor, 1973), WAIS Block Design (Wechsler, 1955), Gollin incomplete Pictures (Gollin, 1960) and there is one which has been designed specifically for use by occupational therapists, the Rivermead Perceptual Assessment Battery (Whiting *et al.* 1984). These tests may be used to identify problems but may need to be supplemented by behavioural observation of, for example, dressing, manoeuvring a wheelchair through a door and face recognition.

Language abilities will similarly affect patients' ability to succeed on verbal memory tasks and on daily life activities involving verbal memory. The patient's ability to communicate functionally should therefore be assessed. It is all too easy for the psychologist or speech therapist to get carried away with the minutiae of speech and language assessment in patients who have 'interesting' dysphasic conditions, whereas what matters clinically is the adequacy of the patient's ability to comprehend auditory and visual verbal instructions, and to communicate with other people. A wide range of aphasia batteries is available in this area, together with additional tests of specific language function. Functional communication skills may be assessed by measures such as the Functional Communication Profile (Sarno, 1969), The Communication Activities in Daily Living Scale (Holland, 1980) and the Speech Questionnaire (Lincoln, 1982). These, rather than the more specific language tests or aphasia batteries, may provide assessments of the effects of language and verbal memory deficits in daily life.

Other aspects of cognitive function which need consideration are speed, attention, reasoning and the ability to inhibit responses. Simple assessments of speed can be made during activities in occupational therapy. For example, the time taken to sort different size sticks, to put pegs in a board or to join dots can easily be recorded. Rating scales can be used to assess whether the patient falls in the average, above or below category and this may be supplemented by more specific assessments of psychomotor reaction time. As a general rule latency measures may show the effects of recovery or treatment long after accuracy measures have stabilized.

Tests of 'frontal lobe' functions may provide valuable information in the context of rehabilitation. Patients with difficulty in initiating or inhibiting responses have in effect a dual deficit which makes their ability to cope with other deficits, such as memory problems, far less than would otherwise be the case. Indeed, such patients often fail on memory and other tests because they fail to carry out an initial analysis of the demands of the situation, and respond impulsively and inappropriately and are then unable to shift from the inappropriate to more appropriate responses.

Mayes (1986) suggests various tests of frontal lobe function which might be incorporated into a complete memory assessment. These include the Wisconsin Card Sorting Test (Milner, 1964) the shorter modified version might also be appropriate (Nelson, 1976), test of verbal and visual fluency (Jones-Gotman and Milner, 1977) and a cognitive estimations test (Shallice and Evans, 1978).

Another crucial predictor of rehabilitation success is the extent to which the patient has any awareness of the nature and severity of his deficit. This may need to be assessed continually throughout the rehabilitation process, and it is here that discrepancies between the patient's assessment of his or her problem and others' assessment of the problem becomes of particular significance. When discrepancies arise, a judicial use of behavioural treatments, individually or group based, and directive counselling with clear behavioural targets may be particularly useful. A group setting in which patients report their assessment of each other may well carry more weight to the patient than the therapist reporting. The group setting may be particularly appropriate for dealing with problems of awareness of deficit (Chapter 9).

Cognitive deficits are striking after acute brain damage, but they comprise only part of the total picture of deficits which include physical as well as affective/behavioural changes. Physical deficits may impose limitations on cognitive ability by reducing the opportunity for interaction with other people, but emotional, behavioural and personality changes may have an

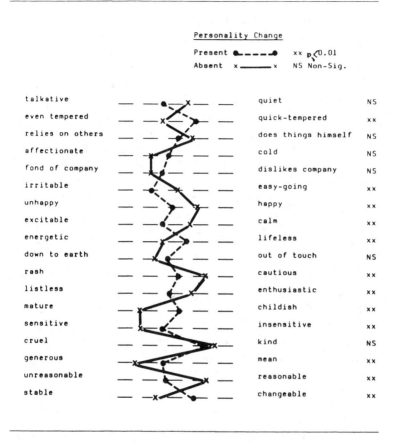

**Figure 2.1** Personality profile and presence of personality change in 55 cases, six months after severe head injury.

even greater impact on the patient's ability to identify and process information in an appropriate way (McKinlay and Brooks *et al.*, 1981; Brooks and McKinlay, 1983). The behavioural and personality changes should therefore be examined as a routine part of the assessment, often using simple and purpose-built tests. An example of such a test is shown in Figure 2.1, which comprises a list of bipolar adjectives used in the identification and assessment of personality changes after severe head injury (Brooks and McKinlay, 1983).

## CONCLUSIONS

Assessment for rehabilitation is more than simply applying a series of standardized tests. Some of the functions which are known to predict rehabilitation and vocational success cannot conveniently be assessed by means of readily available standard measures and the assessment procedure has to be adapted to the problems encountered by the patient and to the different environments in which the patient may find himself. Assessment should include behavioural and interpersonal functioning as well as cognitive and psychomotor functions. All the members of the rehabilitation team should be involved in the assessment of patients and should meet regularly, perhaps weekly, to pool their information. They can then use this pooled information to structure and plan each patient's rehabilitation programme. The programme for each patient should be individually tailored, with short- and long-term goals, which are clearly operationally identified and known to the patient and staff. A rehabilitation regime that simply fits patients into a regular 'unit regime', common to all patients is likely to be less successful than one that institutes a regime derived from a detailed assessment of the particular problems of each patient, and which evaluates the extent to which the goals of the regime have been reached.

## REFERENCES

Albert, M.S., Butters, N. and Levin, J. (1979) Temporal gradients in the retrograde amnesia of patients with alcoholic Korsakoff's disease, *Archives of Neurology*, **36**, 211–16.

Andrews, K. and Stewart, J. (1979) Stroke recovery: he can but does he? *Rheumatology and Rehabilitation*, **18**, 43–8.

Bennett-Levy, J. and Powell, G.E. (1980) The subjective memory questionnaire (SMQ): an investigation in self-reporting of 'real-life' memory skills. *British Journal of Social and Clinical Psychology*, **19**, 177–83.

Benton, A.L. (1950) A multiple choice type of the visual retention test. *Archives Neurology and Psychiatry*, **64**, 699–707.

Benton, A.L. (1974) *The Revised Visual Retention Test*, Psychological Corporation, New York.

Brooks, D.N. (1972) Memory and head injury. *Journal of Nervous Mental Diseases*, **155**, 350–5.

Brooks, D.N. (1975) Long- and short-term memory in head injured patients. *Cortex*, ii, 329–40.

Brooks, D.N. (1976) Wechsler Memory Scale performance and its relationship to brain damage after severe closed head injury. *Journal of Neurology, Neurosurgery and Psychiatry*, **39**, 593–601.

Brooks, D.N. (1979) Psychological deficits after severe blunt head injury: their significance and rehabilitation, in *Research in Psychology in Medicine*, D.J. Obourne, M.M. Gruneberg and J.R. Eisier 2, Academic Press, London, pp. 469–76.

Brooks, D.N. (1983) Disorders of memory, in *Rehabilitation of the Head Injured Patient*, M. Rosenthal, E.R. Griffith, M.R. Bond and G.D. Miller, F.A. Davis Company, Philadelphia.

Brooks, D.N. and Aughton, M.E. (1979) Cognitive recovery during the first year after severe blunt head injury. *International Rehabilitation Medicine*, **1**, 166–72.

Brooks, D.N. and Baddeley, A. (1976) What can amnesiacs learn? *Neuropsychologia*, **14**, 111–22.

Brooks, D.N. and McKinlay, W.W. (1983) Personality and behaviour change after severe blunt head injury: a relative's point of view. *Journal of Neurology, Neurosurgery and Psychiatry*, **46**, 336–44.

Brooks, D.N., Aughton, M.E., Bond, M.R., James, P. and Rizvi, S. (1980) Cognitive sequelae in relationship to early indices of severity of brain damage after severe blunt head injury. *Journal of Neurology, Neurosurgery and Psychiatry*, **43**, 529–34.

Chadwick, O., Rutter, M., Schaffer, D. and Shrout, P.E. (1981) A prospective study of children with head injuries. IV: specific cognitive effects. *Journal of Clinical Neuropsychology*, **3**, 101–20.

Erickson, R.C. and Scott, M.I. (1977) Clinical memory testing: a review. *Psychological Bulletin*, **84**, 1130–49.

Gianutsos, R and Gianutsos, J. (1979) Rehabilitating the verbal recall of brain injured patients by mnemonic training: an experimental demonstration using single case methodology. *Journal of Clinical Neuropsychology*, **1**, 117–35.

Glasgow, R.E., Zeiss, R.A., Barrera, M. and Lewinsohn, P.M. (1977) Case studies on remediating memory deficits in brain damaged individuals. *Journal of Clinical Psychology*, **33**, 1049–54.

Gollin, E.S. (1960) Developmental studies of visual recognition of incomplete objects. *Perceptual and Motor Skills*, **3**, 289–98.

Herrman, D. and Neisser, U. (1978) An inventory of everyday memory experiences. In *Practical Aspects of Memory*, M.M. Gruneberg, P. Morris and R. Sykes, Academic Press, London.

Holland, A.L. (1980) *Communicative Abilities in Daily Living*, University Park Press, Baltimore.

Inglis, J. (1957) An experimental study of learning and memory function in elderly patients. *Journal of Medical Science*, **103**, 798–803.

Jones-Gotman, M. and Milner, B. (1977) Design fluency: the invention of non-sense drawings after focal cortical lesions, *Neuropsychologia*, **15**, 653–74.

Kapur, N. (1987) Some comments on the technical acceptability of

Warrington's Recognition Memory Test, *British Journal of Clinical Psychology*, **26**, 144–46.

Kimura, D. (1963) Right termporal lobe damage. *Archives Neurology*, **8**, 254–71.

Kopelman, M., Wilson, B.A and Baddeley A.D. (1990) *The autobiographical memory interview*, Thames Valley Test Company, Bury, St Edmunds.

Levin, H.S., Grossman, R.G., Sarwar, M. and Meyers, C.A. (1981) Linguistic recovery after closed head injury. *Brain and Language*, **12**, 360–74.

Lewinsohn, P.M. and Graf, M. (1973) A follow-up study of persons referred for vocational rehabilitation who have suffered brain injury. *Journal of Community Psychology*, **1**, 57–62.

Lincoln, N.B. (1981) Discrepancies between capabilities and performance of activities of daily living in multiple sclerosis patients. *International Rehabilitation Medicine*, **3**, 84–8.

Lincoln, N.B. (1982) The Speech Questionnaire: and assessment of functional language ability. *International Rehabilitiation Medicine*, **4**, 114–17.

Lincoln, N.B. and Staples, D. (1987) A maze learning test for the assessment of memory with physically disabled patients, *Clinical Rehabilitation*, **1**, 197–202.

Lincoln, N.B. and Tinson, D.J. (1989) The relation between subjective and objective memory impairment after stroke, *British Journal of Clinical Psychology*, **28**, 61–5.

Loring, D.W. and Papanicolaou, A.C. (1987) Memory assessment in neuropsychology: Theoretical considerations and practical viability, *Journal of Clinical and Experimental Neuropsychology*, **9**, 340–58.

McKinlay, W.W. and Brooks, D.N. (1984) Methodological problems in assessing psychosocial recovery following severe head injury, *Journal of Clinical Neuropsychology*, **6**, 87–100.

McKinlay, W.W, Brooks, D.N., Bond, M.R. *et al.* (1981) The short-term outcome of severe blunt head injury as reported by the relatives of the injured person. *Journal Neurol. Neuro-Surgery and Psychiatry*, **44**, 527–33.

Mayes, A.R. (1986) Learning and memory disorders and their assessment, *Neuropsychologia*, **24**, 25–39.

Milner, B. (1964) Some effects of frontal lobectomy in man, in *The Frontal Granular Cortex and Behaviour*, J.M. Warren and K. Akert (Eds), McGraw-Hill, New York. 313–34.

Nelson, H. (1976) A modified card sorting test sensitive to frontal lobe deficits. *Cortex*, **12**, 313–24.

Nelson, H. (1982) *National Adult Reading Test*, NFER-Nelson, Windsor.

Parkin, A.J. (1987) *Memory and Amnesia*, Blackwell, Oxford.

Parker, S.A. and Serrats, A.P. (1976) Memory recovery after traumatic coma. *Acta Neurochir*, **34**, 71–7.

Prigatano, G.P. (1978) Wechsler Memory Scale: A selective review of the literature, *Journal of Clinical Psychology*, **34**, 816–32.

Raven, J.C. (1958) *Mill Hill Vocabulary Scale*, 2nd edn., Lewis and Co., London.

Rey, A. (1959) *Le test de coupe de figure complexe*, Editions Centre de Psychologie Appliquee, Paris.

Sarno, M.T. (1969) *The Functional Communications Profile: Manual of Directions*, Institute of Rehabilitation Medicine, New York University Medical Centre.

Shallice, T. and Evans, M.E. (1978) The involvement of the frontal lobes in cognitive estimation, *Cortex*, **14**, 294–303.

Sunderland, A., Harris, J. and Baddeley, A.D. (1983) Do laboratory tests predict everyday memory? A neuropsychological study. *Journal of Verbal Learning and Verbal Behaviour*, **22**, 341–57.

Tinson, D.J. and Lincoln, N.D. (1987) Subjective memory impairment after stroke. *International Disability Studies*, **9**, 6–9.

van Zomeren, A.H., Brouwer, W.H. and Deelman, B.G. (1983) Attentional deficits: the riddles of selectivity, speed and alertness. in *Closed Head Injury: Social, Psychological and Family Consequences*, D.N. Brooks, ed, Oxford University Press, Oxford.

Walton, D. and Black, D.A. (1957) The validity of a psychological test of brain damage. *British Journal of Medical Psychology*, **30**, 270–9.

Warrington, E.K. (1971) Perception of naturalistic stimuli in patients with focal brain lesions. *Journal of Brain Research*, **31**, 370.

Warrington, E.K. (1974) Deficient recognition memory in organic amnesia. *Cortex*, **10**, 284–91.

Warrington, E.K. (1984) *Recognition Memory Test*, NFER-Nelson, Windsor.

Warrington, E.K. and James, M. (1967) Disorders of visual perception in patients with localised cerebral lesions. *Neuropsychologia*, **5**, 1–13.

Warrington, E.K. and Taylor, A.M. (1973) The contribution of the right parietal lobe to object recognition. *Cortex*, **7**, 152–64.

Wechsler, D. (1945) A standardised memory scale for clinical use. *Journal of Psychology*, **19**, 87–95.

Wechsler, D. (1955) *Wechsler Adult Intelligence Scale*, Psychological Corporation, New York.

Wechsler, D. (1981) Wechsler Adult Intelligence Scale – Revised. Psychological Corporation, Harcourt Brace Jovanovich, New York.

Wechsler, D. (1987) Wechsler Memory Scale – Revised. Psychological Corporation, Harcourt Brace Jovanovich, New York.

Whiting, S., Lincoln, N.B., Bhavani G. *et al.* (1984) *The Rivermead Perceptual Assessment Battery*, NFER – Nelson, Windsor.

Williams, M. (1968) The measurement of memory in clinical practice. *British Journal of Social and Clinical Psychology*, **7**, 19–34.

Wilson, B. (1982) Success and failure in memory training following a cerebral vascular accident. *Cortex*, **18**, 581–94.

Wilson, B.A. (1988) Assessing everyday memory, in MRC News, June 1988.

Wilson, B.A. Assessment of memory in (ed. Beech, J. and Harding, L.) *Psychological Assessment*, NFER – Nelson, Windsor (in press).

Wilson, B.A., Cockburn, J. and Baddeley, A. (1985) *Rivermead Behavioural Memory Test*, Thames Valley Test Company, Bury St Edmunds, England. 46–51.

Wilson, B.A. and Cockburn, J. (1988) The Prices Test: a simple test of retrograde amnesia, in Gruneberg, M., Morris, P.E. and Sykes, R. *Practical Aspects of Memory*, Wiley, Chichester.

Wilson, J.T.L., Brooks, D.N. and Phillips, W.A. (1982) Using a microcomputer to study perception, memory and attention after head injury. Paper presented at *Fifth Annual Conference of International Neuropsychological Society*, June 15–18, Deauville, France.

# Chapter 3

# Ways to help memory∗†
## JOHN E. HARRIS

### INTRODUCTION

Several recent books and papers on memory have noted the passing of 100 years of memory research, taking 1885 as the starting date when Ebbinghaus published his experimental studies of memory. The study of memory has continued on a large scale and in recent times hundreds of research papers have been published each year.

With all this research, you might expect that sophisticated ways of improving memory would be available by now, or at least be in the final stages of development. However, most of the work has been on how things are forgotten; very little has been connected with methods of improving memory. Among the reasons for this is the limited number of approaches that seemed to be available. The research that did appear from time to time was often superficial in approach, doing little more than testing whether a technique worked or not. Improvements to techniques seemed more likely to come from a better understanding of memory processes, the object of most memory research.

Remembering techniques have also had a tarnished image among researchers. This comes from the way remembering techniques have been used for sensational entertainments

∗ This chapter was written early in 1988. Between then and publication, there have been important technological developments and new products in the area of personal organizers, from pocket sized hardware to new pc software.
† Editor's note: There is an up-to-date memory aids catalogue available from Dr Narinder Kapur, Memory Aids Unit, Wessex Neurological Centre, Southampton General Hospital, Southampton SO9 4XY. This gives detailed information and prices of new products in this field.

and the crude commercialism so often associated with selling ways to improve your memory. You may have seen advertisements in the press headed 'Is memory your problem?' or 'Develop a super-power memory'.

In the past, academic psychologists, with their scientific aspirations, have often preferred pure to applied research, and their wish to avoid being associated with sensational commercialism may have further inhibited research on memory aids.

With the recent pressure for academics to be more application conscious and commercially minded, there is a little more interest in memory aids. Examples are symposia on memory aids at memory conferences, and Gruneberg's (1987) adaptation of traditional word association techniques to remembering new words when learning foreign languages. However, reaction of fellow psychologists to Gruneberg's linkword method and to his controversial appearance on a popular TV show, *The Magic of Memory* (Daniels, 1988), shows that academic opinion is still divided over the desirability of such applications.

Even Gruneberg's methods are developments of traditional word-association techniques, and his degree of interest is unusual. So this chapter does not catalogue a series of super new mnemonics that are being developed in psychological laboratories. Rather its purposes are to explain the broad categories of existing ways of improving memory as shown in Figure 3.1, and to discuss reminders to do things, an area where there are current developments, though these come more from the fields of electronics and computing than from psychology.

## INTERNAL STRATEGIES

### Naturally learned internal strategies

I shall start with the naturally learned strategies, because they are rather different from the others; they are strategies most of us use quite naturally, often without realizing it. Imagine that you are asked to memorize 20 historical dates in five minutes; then you are tested and get, say, 14 right. If you are now given another five minutes to improve your performance as

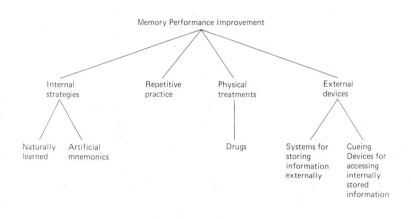

Figure 3.1 Ways of improving memory as set out in this chapter.

much as possible, how would you split your time among the dates? Most adults would concentrate more time on those dates they had got wrong in the first test.

You might think this is an obvious strategy. After all, it is a waste of time trying to memorize something you have already learnt. But developmental psychologists investigating how children learn to use their memories efficiently have shown that young children do not use this type of strategy. For example, a study at the University of Minnesota (Masur, McIntyre and Flavell, 1973) showed that this particular strategy does not appear until the age of seven to nine years.

Another example that is familiar to experimental psychologists is the strategy, often used in the free recall of a randomly ordered word list, that leads to the last presented items being recalled first. We all use a great many of these natural memory strategies, but they are not normally thought of as memory *aids*, because they are so much part of our normal memory skills.

### Artificial mnemonics

The other group of internal strategies often go by the name 'mnemonics' (though some people use this term for anything that improves memory). These skills are similar to the ones that I have just described, except that they have to be consciously learned and used, often requiring considerable effort. Consequently, most of us seldom use them, even when we are fully mature adults (Harris, 1980). However, they do form the main content of most books and courses on memory improvement. So what are they and do they work?

Most of these techniques are variations on a very few themes, perhaps not more than a dozen. I shall describe some examples. One technique that can be used to remember a random sequence of words, maintaining the order, is to make up a story connecting them. You can then retell the story to yourself when you need to remember the words. This technique has been shown to be effective in the psychological laboratory (Bower and Clark, 1969), but how often do you want to remember a list of words? You may reply that you frequently want to remember a list of things to buy on a shopping trip. But for this purpose most people prefer to use external aids, such as a shopping list. This preference came out clearly in interview studies I carried out, first with Southampton University students and then with a group of Cambridge women, who were mainly homemakers (Harris, 1980).

Another mnemonic helps you recognize people's faces and to remember their names. First you study the person's face to find an unusual feature. Next you change their name into something meaningful, and finally you associate the two with a ridiculous image. For example, red-bearded Mr Hills could be imagined with hills growing out of his beard.

Even if this works in the laboratory, how useful is it in the real world? One could argue that on meeting people for the first time we are usually expected to strike up a conversation with them. This does not leave much time for finding unusual features of their faces or even meaningful aspects of their names. Anyway, most people do not have convenient red beards!

For most of us learning things this way demands a considerable effort, more effort than we are usually prepared
to make unless we are having unusual difficulty, or have
a professional need to remember names or similar information. For example, salesmen and professionals such as
solicitors may need to know the names of at least their
regular customers or clients. The magician and TV show
presenter, Paul Daniels (1988), explained on *The Magic of
Memory* programme that he uses mnemonics frequently in
his work; it looks unprofessional to forget, for example, the
names of volunteers from the audience who help with his
magic.

This and similar techniques may also be of some use
in helping people with certain types of memory problem
to learn the names, for example, of their workmates or
rehabilitation staff, when the problem may be learning the
names at all, rather than learning them on the first meeting
(Wilson and Moffat, 1984).

For the rest of us, we usually learn names over the first
few times we meet people, though we may well make use of
business cards, or notice and remember that the name is the
same or similar to one we already know, without recognizing
that we are using any sort of aid.

A third type of mnemonic is exemplified by the sentence
'Richard Of York Gained Battles In Vain'. The first letters of
the words in this sentence are also the first letters of the
colours of the rainbow, and they are in order: Red, Orange,
Yellow, Green, Blue, Indigo, Violet.

First letter mnemonics are mainly useful when you need to
remember things in their correct order, and then only when
you do not prefer to write them down. I can only think of two
such occasions. The first is when the items and the order
they occur in are permanent, and when you may want to
refer to them, in order, from time to time. The order of the
colours of the rainbow and of the cranial nerves are good
examples. This is also true of rhymes we use to help us
remember facts, such as the one that starts, 'Thirty days
hath September . . .' The facts are also permanent. More
typical of the things we have difficulty remembering in
everyday life are the items on a shopping list, which may
vary from one shopping trip to another, so that it is hardly

worth learning a new version of the mnemonic on each occasion.

For the patient with memory deficits, however, their most fundamental difficulties may be associated with retaining relatively stable information such as common routes, addresses, names of colleagues, or hospital staff, and various types of sequences. In such cases mnemonics may well help.

The second situation in which first-letter and rhyme mnemonics are useful is when written reminders are not available. In examinations written reminders are normally forbidden, regarded as a form of cheating. Learned mnemonics, on the other hand, are usually acceptable, and anyway the invigilator cannot see them! Certainly students do use mnemonics, particularly the first letter and rhymes varieties (though according to my study, Harris 1980, even students use these mnemonics much less often than they use external aids, such as diaries, memos, shopping lists and asking someone for a reminder).

Patients with memory problems may find themselves in a similar situation if they do not wish to be seen using external aids, such as written reminders, which might mark them out as handicapped.

If readers want to find out more about mnemonics, I suggest they consult Higbee (1977), Lorayne and Lucas (1975), Morris (1977) and Yates (1966).

### REPETITIVE PRACTICE

Repeated practice is a method we frequently use for a wide range of learning and memorizing, from children memorizing the alphabet and their multiplication tables and actors learning their lines, to the learning of motor skills, such as driving, riding a bike, or playing a game such as football. Indeed this is the normal way we acquire skills. Two important factors to consider are how to make practice efficient and whether practice is always applied in appropriate circumstances.

A classical finding in psychology is that practice distributed widely over time is more effective than the same amount of practice fitted into a short period. This has been found on many types of learning and with comparisons over different ranges of time.

When we are learning by practice, it is usually helpful to know how we are doing, and many sorts of practice involve feedback of results. If learning involves a series of recall attempts or trials, it is better to arrange them so that attempts tend to be correct and lead to positive reinforcement and encouragement than to make them so difficult that many are incorrect.

Landauer and Bjork (1978) and Baddeley (1982, and see chapter 1) have combined the advantages of distributed practice and correct recall attempts into a method of initially testing after a very short interval and gradually increasing it, only shortening it again if the learner makes an error. This can be a very effective strategy.

Although in some dramatic, and thankfully rare, syndromes even repeated practice is of little benefit, memory problems often mean that patients need practice to remember things they would otherwise have learnt without. In these cases, the normal principles will usually apply to practice, such as the Landauer and Bjork technique being effective.

Although repeated practice can often lead to high levels of learning, we need to be cautious about using it on memory games such as Kim's game or on laboratory tasks such as paired-associate learning. A survey of the management of memory disorders in Britain (Harris and Sunderland, 1981) showed that such techniques were in widespread use in rehabilitation units. However, it is not at all clear that they are effective. If the practice is applied to a task or material that the patient needs to learn, then it can clearly be of benefit, but the tasks are often artificial or based on games. Their use appears to be

> based on the assumption that memory responds like a 'mental muscle', and that exercising it on one task will strengthen it for use on other tasks, so that any improvement on artificial games will generalize to the requirements of everyday life. Such a view seems too simple and over-optimistic. Current theoretical views about memory, although diverse, tend to agree that memory represents a far more complicated set of interacting cognitive skills

and abilities than any idea of a mental muscle seems to imply. More damaging is the evidence that memory skills acquired with practice on very specific tasks may not generalize even to apparently similar tasks. For example, Ericsson, Chase and Falcon (1980) trained a student in conventional digit span tests. Over 20 months his span increased from about 7 to 80 digits; however, the effect of the practice did not even generalize to memory span for consonants, which remained at only about 6 when digit span had already increased substantially.

However, there are also arguments in support of repetitive practice on games or laboratory tasks. First, it may be good for the patients' morale, because he knows something is being done to help his memory problems, and he will also be aware of his improvements on the tasks he is practising. This may encourage him that it is possible to improve his performance, so that he feels it is worth making an effort with everyday memory tasks. Second, there is some evidence, from animal studies, of neural regeneration following brain injury (Wall, 1975), and also that early intervention with physical exercise promotes recovery after motor cortex damage better than later intervention (Black, Markowitz and Cianci, 1975). It is at least possible that mental exercise during a critical period of neural regeneration may in some way enhance the regeneration. (Harris and Sunderland, 1981, p. 208)

If this turns out to be the case, it throws into question the common practice of waiting for a stable baseline before intervening with memory training, a practice that derives from the need for assessment rather than the prime objective of rehabilitation.

## PHYSICAL TREATMENTS

By physical treatments I mean ways of directly manipulating the basic biological and chemical processes on which memory depends or that represent memory at a physiological level. Certainly these processes can be influenced, as studies of the effects of drugs on memory have shown, and first-hand knowledge of the effect that alcohol can have on memory is not confined to psychologists and scientists!

Most of the experimental work has been done with drugs that, like alcohol, decrease memory performance. They are often used, as in the case of hyoscine, in an effort to stimulate in normal people components of clinical syndromes, such as Alzheimer's disease. This is done in order to understand which aspects of the physiological changes produce the memory deficits associated with the disorders. Sometimes the effects of these drugs has been lessened by others, such as piracetam or physostigmine, that have a counter effect (Kopelman, 1986). By extention, this second group has been tried as a therapy for Alzheimer patients with some limited success; there have even been reported benefits to normal young subjects (Davis, Mohs and Tinklenberg, 1978; Sitaram, Weingartner and Gillin, 1978). This topic is covered in more detail in Chapter 7 by Michael Kopelman, so I shall move on to the next type of aid.

## EXTERNAL METHODS

The last main category is external methods, such as the traditional knotted handkerchief. The spontaneous use of external methods to remember things develops during childhood, just as the use of internal ones does.

In one study Kreutzer, Leonard and Flavell (1975) questioned children about various aspects of memory; for example, they asked them how many ways they could think of to be sure they would take their skates to school the next day. The children gave more external methods than internal ones, such as putting their skates by the front door, putting them in their satchels, or asking someone to remind them. This was true for all four age groups, whose ages ranged from 6 to 11 years, but the older groups had much richer repertoires of external methods than did the younger ones.

The researchers found a similar result with another question about methods of remembering a friend's birthday party, and one about a friend trying to work out the age of his dog; they were asked what he could do to help him remember which Christmas he had received the dog as a puppy. Again all the groups of children gave many more external methods than internal ones, and the older children had richer repertoires.

## External information storage

External aids can be divided into two groups. One group is made up of those aids that we use to store information externally. We may use them either because they are more accurate or complete than internal storage, or because internal storage mechanisms may be overloaded. Sometimes it involves storing small amounts of information over short periods of time, such as jotting down intermediate results during mental calculations; or it may involve storage of large quantities of information over much longer periods. Examples of this are the information stored in documents, filing systems, books, libraries and, of course, computers.

Professor Hunter (1979) of Keele University referred to these systems as 'communal memory stores' and he noted that their functions include the passing of knowledge from generation to generation, in effect a kind of cultural memory. (He also pointed out that the technology and culture of non-literate societies are remembered with aids such as rituals. The example he quoted from Dr Bronowski was a ritual that ensures that the different stages of making a sword are all performed correctly and in the right order. Chanting and recitation can also be used as cultural memory aids, the younger individuals slowly learning the chants and words, and gradually becoming able to join in and take over.)

The latest type of external memory store is provided by computers. In fact, it is in this role that computers have had the biggest impact on most people. Details of their bank accounts, car registration, mortgages, pay and tax are all likely to be stored in computer files. This concept of storing vast quantities of organized information that can be accessed very rapidly is familiar to most of us, but for personal use, things are moving much more slowly, with the cost often difficult to justify except in the workplace. There are still very few personal users of Prestel apart from computer hobbyists and although laser discs are appearing that contain encyclopaedias, census information and so on, they're still expensive ways of gaining access to vast communal memory aids.

External storage in the form of written information, such as timetables, lists, plans, sketchmaps and diagrams can be a very cheap and effective way of helping people with memory deficits. Although this may be seen as a 'crutch' rather than a method of memorizing the information, it can overcome the practical difficulties and allow the patient to lead a more normal life. Also, in some cases, repeated use of such an aid is likely to lead to some of the information being memorized.

For patients unable to read written information, an alternative is to use pocket memo recorders or dictating machines. However, they are not as flexible in the ways they can be used and patients may have difficulty operating them.

Some written aids, such as shopping lists, only store relatively small amounts of information, acting as cues for actions that also require the use of internally stored information. The next section covers such cueing aids.

## CUEING DEVICES

This section on cueing devices is longer than the others, firstly because remembering to do things has been a personal interest of mine (Harris, 1984; Harris and Wilkins, 1982), and secondly because, unlike the case with mnemonics, there is a lack of alternative sources.

The properties needed in cueing aids are very different from mere storage of information. For example, the words 'wedding anniversary' in a diary are usually sufficient (if they are read at the appropriate time), because you are quite capable of retrieving from your own memory the information that you should buy a card or take whatever action is appropriate. What you need is a *cue* for a particular action, not a detailed description of the action itself.

Cueing devices vary in the type of cue they provide. An alarm cooking-timer provides an *active* reminder, while a shopping list provides *specific* information about which items to buy. This variation points to criteria for the effectiveness of cueing devices and the cues they provide.

For a cue to have the best chance of being effective it needs to have certain properties. First, it should be given as close as possible before the time when the action is required – being reminded as you leave home in the morning to buy some bread on the way home still leaves plenty of time to forget. Secondly, it should be active rather than passive – a passive reminder in a diary may fail if you forget to consult it. Thirdly, it should be a specific reminder for the particular action that is required – a knotted handkerchief may only remind you that something must be remembered, but not what that something is.

So an ideal cueing aid might whisper discreetly in your ear, just at the right moment, what you should do. Human helpers can do this, and it can be a useful strategy for forgetful people to learn to ask others to remind them – if they choose someone reliable! As yet there isn't any artificial device that can provide such a whisper and some sort of compromise has to be made.

Normal people vary a great deal in how they organize their lives, what sort of things they have to remember to do, how easily they remember without external aids and which aids they find helpful and convenient. For people with clinical memory problems you have to add the variation in type and severity of the problems. Any particular sort of aid may only be of use in a tiny proportion of clinical cases.

Also memory problems are usually associated with learning difficulties, which may be simply a different view of the same problem – from the opposite end of the retention interval. As a result, people with memory problems may find it more difficult to learn to use complicated hi-tech aids, which are too often designed by people who know about the technological side, but not about how to make things easy to use. So it is not possible to prescribe memory aid X for memory problem Y, rather the clinician or therapist needs to fit the aid to the individual patient, if one is suitable at all. In what follows I use examples to point out important issues to consider in choosing cueing memory aids for particular purposes.

### Active cues

Traditional diaries, even in their expensive and fashionable form as executive organizers like Filofax, are not active. They

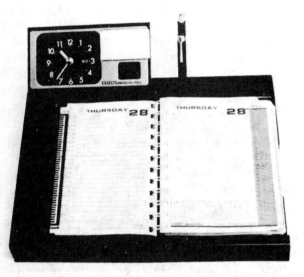

**Figure 3.2** Esselte 'Electronic Diary'.

rely on the user consulting them regularly. This can still be very effective for a well-organized person who, for example, consults the diary in the morning and then makes a mental plan of the day's activities. But there are plenty of situations when it can fail, such as for someone whose days are mostly alike and who only has the occasional appointment in a diary; they are unlikely to consult it often enough for it to be effective. Even people who have memorized a plan for the day may rely on the finishing of one activity to make them think about the next; if one activity overruns they may forget the next until too late.

The Esselte 'Electronic Diary' shown in Figure 3.2 is like a desk diary with a built-in alarm. It consists of an alarm clock and a pad of paper printed in the form of a diary. Each page is divided into quarter-hour sections, opposite which you can write *specific* reminder messages. Then you use the same ordinary lead pencil to join two lines of electrically conducting ink, opposite the time you require the reminder. The graphite in the pencil mark completes the circuit and the alarm rings at the time indicated. When this happens, you find out the current time by looking at the clock, and you can then tell what you are supposed to be doing by reading what is written opposite this time on the pad.

## Timely cues

The Esselte Electronic Diary is a very neat idea and should work well for someone confined within earshot of the alarm, such as in an office or laboratory, provided that the action being cued can be performed straight away at the quarter-hour times at which the alarm can be set. You only need a few minutes, or sometimes seconds, to forget. I once set an Esselte alarm for 2.45pm to remind me of a meeting ten minutes later. To fill this ten-minute wait I picked up an article to read. Fifteen minutes later I was still reading the article! In later research (Harris and Wilkins, 1982), we found that people can forget to do things in ten seconds or less, if they are distracted by, say, watching an exciting film.

## Specific cues

Alarm watches and clocks are, of course, active and you can often set them to the minute, and some allow you to set multiple alarms up to a year in advance. But imagine setting one to ring at three o'clock on a day ten months from now. Would you remember then why you had set it? With several alarms set for each week, you might have difficulty in much less than ten months, especially if you suffer from a memory impairment.

Some watch alarms attempt to deal with specificity. Typically four different signals can be set independently. Each alarm consists of a group of 'pips', so that one goes 'pip . . . pip . . . pip', the second goes 'pip pip . . . pip pip . . . pip pip', and so on. At first, this seems to be a rea-sonable way to provide specificity, and it might be useful for a patient who has difficulty remembering a limited number of regular actions so that an association can be learned between a particular signal and the required action,

(though a mnemonic may be needed to learn the association). For more general use with the variety of things
we normally want to remember to do, there's a problem
with such an arbitrary form of specificity, in that you
have to remember the relevance of each signal on each
occasion you use it, or you have to write it down somewhere.

The Esselte Electronic Diary wins again, as it allows you to
write a conventional diary entry. So if instead of withdrawing
it altogether, Esselte had produced a version with alarm
settings at minute rather than quarter-hour intervals, would
they have had a winner on their hands? Unfortunately, there
is more to it than just producing active, timely and specific
cues – the machine has to be convenient, easy and available
to use.

### Portability and general utility

To be available when we want to use it, an aid has to be
carried around with us, and whether we do this depends
mainly on the balance of its usefulness and the hassle of
carrying it around.

This is illustrated by alarm watches; although most do not
give specific cues, they do have two advantages over aids
such as cooking timers. First they are very portable and,
secondly, they have another, more frequent use – they tell
the time. As a result watches are normally carried around,
so you do not have to remember separately to take them with
you when you want to use them.

The trade-off between utility and portability is illustrated
with conventional diaries; bigger ones may have more room
and supplementary information and so may be more useful,
but small ones are easier to carry around. The convenience
cost of carrying a large one depends on whether you use a
large handbag or briefcase, wear a jacket with big pockets
or just trousers with small ones and so on. The benefits of
a large one might extend beyond its contents to impressing
people with a leather-bound Filofax!

So to be available when we need to use them, cueing
devices should be portable and of use in as many ways as
possible.

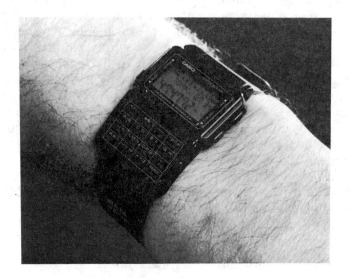

**Figure 3.3** Casio 'Data Bank Watch'.

## Capacity: number and length of cues

We are gradually moving towards electronic diaries from precursors such as alarm watches, calculators with alarm facilities and scheduling programs on personal and portable computers. Already we have the Casio Data Bank Watch in Figure 3.3, which allows you to key in a reminder message to go with the alarms (costing about £27 at time of writing). The message is displayed when the alarm sounds. Although you can enter reminders for up to a year ahead, you are limited to 50 appointments or an average 1 per week (less if you also use its facility for storing phone numbers). After using a Data Bank watch for six months, Moss (1986) reviewed it very positively, the reminder function in particular. Although still enthusiatic after a further nine months, he still used a conventional diary as well. If such devices are developed to the stage where they replace ordinary diaries, they will need far greater capacity.

Long cues are not usually necessary for people with normal memories, especially for reminders in the next few days. When colleagues used the Esselte Electronic Diary for a few days each, all their reminders were much shorter than would fit on the line, only one being as long as four words. We have already considered the power of the short cue 'wedding anniversary' and many others can be as short – consider 'buy bread', 'fetch children', 'lunch with Anne', 'club meeting', 'dentist', 'car service'. Over short periods we seldom need more than three words and even these can sometimes be abbreviated. Over longer periods some cues need to be slightly longer and more explicit, such as *take children to dentist* or *ring travel agent about air tickets*.

The capacity of some cueing aids to store reminder messages is assigned so that a fixed amount, say 40 characters, is available for each reminder; the space not used is not made available for other messages. A better arrangement is for the reminder simply to use as much of the total capacity as is necessary, but no more. This allows an occasional longer message to be used without wasting the same amount of space on all the others. Longer messages are more important for people with certain sorts of memory problem.

Some memory aids allow supplementary information to be stored separately from the cueing information, such as telephone numbers in the Data Bank Watch. However, this has more to do with storing information externally than with cueing.

### Time range

At present the functions of reminder alarm systems and diaries remain largely separate. We usually set alarms to go off in the next few days, but expect diaries to last a full year. As they become more combined we shall expect to set alarms with diary entries several months ahead and a year will become a reasonable minimum standard.

Whereas the conventional diary year is fixed, so that during December we may need to carry the next year's diary as well, electronic ones could always give us 12 months from today, though this often means deleting past entries to make future days available. It is sometimes useful to review past appointments and reminders, so in moving to electronic diaries we need to consider when and

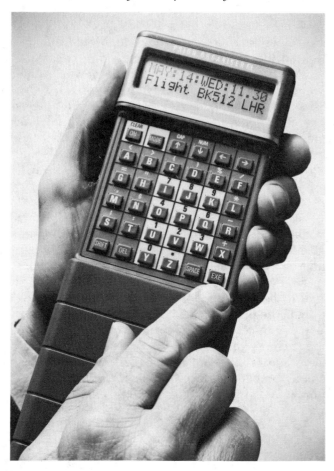

**Figure 3.4** The Psion Organiser II.

how past entries are deleted or overwritten with future ones.

### Searching, reviewing, editing, copying and repeating

If we are setting cues far ahead we need to be able to find, review and sometimes to edit or change them, just as we do with entries in an appointment book. You need to be able to deal with re-scheduled meetings, check you have entered an appointment with, for example, the optician, or find a free two-hour period one afternoon next week to visit someone. It's with this sort of requirement that currently available electronic systems vary considerably.

An example is the Psion Organiser II (Figure 3.4), which is a pocket computer. When I used one for a short period, it impressed me as a very low-cost, hand-held computer, but not as an organizer! Time (years 1900 to 2000) is arranged into half-hour slots, with the display showing the contents of just one slot. This would be fine if appointments came in neat multiples of clock half-hours! Pressing up or down cursor keys takes you back or forwards half-an-hour, while pressing left or right cursor keys takes you back or forward exactly one day. The top line of 16 characters displays the time and date (not the year) and the bottom 16 characters are for displaying a message (longer messages automatically scroll horizontally).

You can find entries by:

1. entering a date and time
2. searching nearby slots with the cursor keys
3. viewing all entries one after the other, chronologically from the first entry after current time until the furthest one in the future
4. searching for a specified string of characters (letters or numbers) in an entry, (e.g. FIND dentist).

This is better than is offered on many devices, but it still lacks a convenient way of finding, say, which afternoons next week have no appointments arranged. You need some form of overview summary or calendar, showing you much longer periods than half an hour, preferably a week or a month, on which previously entered appointments show up.

Such a function exists on Cambridge Computer's Z88 portable computer (Figure 3.5), though it only identifies days in the month that have an entry, without showing even whether it's in the morning or afternoon. It has diary, calendar, clock and alarm facilities that show the beginnings of better design of these functions, but these facilities are not fully integrated with each other. The alarm times (and messages that accompany them) have to be entered quite separately from the diary entries.

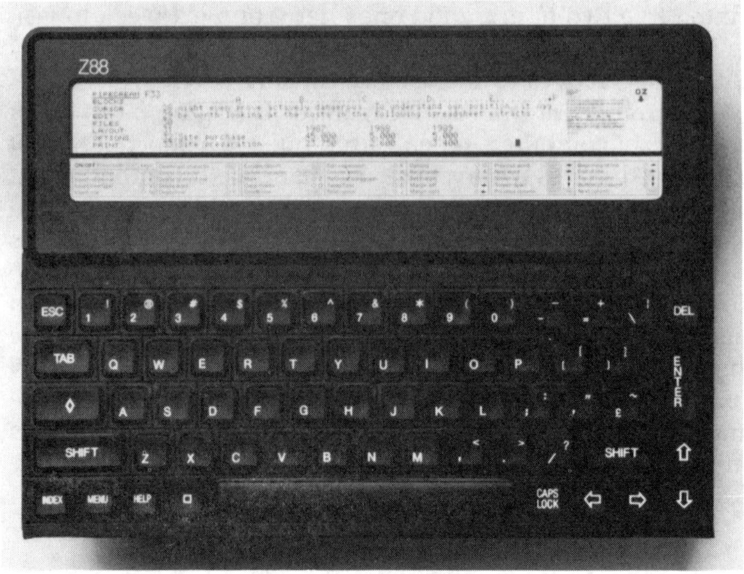

**Figure 3.5** The Cambridge Computer Z88.

On the Z88, these alarms can be made to repeat over a full range of intervals from seconds to years. This sort of repetition can be useful for things such as:

1. remembering anniversaries
2. reminding patients of meal times each day
3. reminding different types of patients of things they need to do regularly, such as taking medicine, doing exercises, swallowing saliva, adjusting posture, going to the lavatory
4. developing new habits.

A related but more general function in the diary facility is the ability to treat an appointment in a diary in the same way as a block of text in a word processor, so that it can easily be copied or moved to another time and/or date without having to retype it.

## Fexible time setting

Often we want to set reminders using the *time elapsed* from now rather than a precise time and date. Examples are wanting a reminder in an hour's time from now or booking an appointment for six weeks from now without having to work out what the date or time will be then. Some alarm watches allow you to set this type of alarm, but often only for 9 or 23 hours ahead. More sophisticated systems could allow you to enter a time-elapsed interval and would then display the time and date at the end of the interval.

## Easy to use

Clearly, if people with clinical memory problems are going to use these sorts of devices, they must be easy to use and it's probable that those currently available will be of significant help to only a very few patients. It's difficult to define for potential buyers all the features that would make cueing aids easy to use and I have covered some already. What is clear is that some aids are unnecessarily difficult to use; designers of such systems too often ignore even elementary aspects of the user interface, particularly where the selling point is the size of the hardware or the low price of the system. The Mind Reader, described in the first edition of this book, on the other hand, made good use of default options to ease the user's task; for example, when setting the date you were first offered 'today' on the display, if the reminder was indeed for today, you only had to press the 'yes' key to set the date.

In the first edition I also mentioned the Toshiba Memo Note II and the Sharp EL-6200 Schedule Planner which functioned in a very similar way to the Casio Data Bank Watch (one of them even gave a monthly overview of appointments). Barbara Wilson (Wilson and Moffat, 1984) used the Memo Note 60 (similar in operation but larger than the Memo Note II) with patients. It takes even normal people a while to learn how to enter the reminders into these machines and Wilson found that this was a great problem for those with memory impairment. Even if this is done for them, some patients cannot remember simple steps such as how to clear the display.

However, from the enquiries I get it is clear some clinicians and therapists do regard this sort of aid as useful with some patients. Although the Sharp and Casio are no longer available, similar calculator-type ones are available costing less than £20; they are smaller (not much bigger than credit cards), with much larger memories for storing more cues with longer messages, and some have larger displays. However, the one I have tried is no easier to use and came with a poor quality user guide. They include the Uni-Com Datacard 4000 (see Figure 3.6), the Super Directory and the Megalogic PD 8000 Pocket Computer (which are similar, but with more memory and a display of 40 characters rather than 20). Devices like these are advertised in mail order booklets that come with credit card bills and Sunday papers. But beware; some have irritating features; on the Datacard you can't change or correct, say, the month, without re-entering the day of the month, the hour and the minute, even though these may be correct.

### Future developments

It's difficult to predict the way cueing aids and diaries will develop, but several trends are clear. First, with highly portable aids, calculator size and smaller, the development effort often goes into the hardware technology and miniaturization. I have come across some horrors in user interface aspects, such as unsuitable ways of mapping basic functions on to keys. On the whole, the larger corporations do not make quite such bad mistakes, but even they have some way to go making these products easier to use.

In personal computers, we are beginning to see sophisticated software that has benefited from experience and feedback from other sorts of personal software (such as word processors). Borland International's 'SideKick Plus' contains a number of useful personal tools, including a 'Time Planner' that contains many of the features I have mentioned. There's a calendar you can call to the screen and use to look at six weeks at a time; you can highlight a date and press RETURN to zoom in on the day's entries, whose start and length can be set to the minute. When the entry times arrive, alarms can be sounded, telephone numbers can be dialled, or a reminder

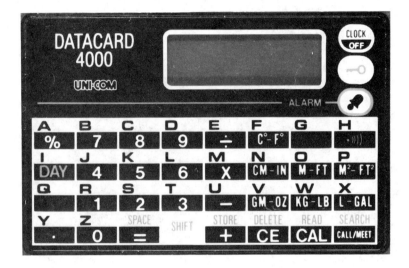

**Figure 3.6** Unicom 'Datacard' 4000.

message can appear on the screen. A separate display can show a summary of up to four weeks, with times when you are busy blocked out, so it's easy to see when you are free. Also a separate facility allows you to search for strings of characters used in an entry or even for vacant time slots of a particular length.

The designers of Lotus 'Agenda' (not due in the UK for three months at time of writing) have allowed the user to enter phrases like 'this afternoon', 'last Mon in Aug' or 'in two days'. Agenda entries can be attached to one or more categories that you can create at any time, and these categories can then be used to present a different *view* of the entries. For example, you could decide to categorize entries on a basis of priority, using high, medium and low; you could then view your entries ordered according to their level of priority. You could also categorize according to the area of your life concerned (job, domestic, charity work and so on) and the type of action required (meetings, reminders to make phone calls, social events, deadlines and so on).

The facilities of both SideKick Plus and Agenda offer a new level of sophistication and adaptability and it may take a generation or two of such programs before they are presented in a way that's easy to use.

Software companies seem to be realizing that 'personal organizers' and 'information managers' are an untapped market and many other programs will be available by the time this book is published. Some names to look for are 'Who/What/When' from Chronos Software, 'Grandview' from Symantec's Living Videotext Division and 'Info-XL' from Valor Software, though at the time of writing I cannot tell you any more about them.

We have seen enormous strides in many areas of personal software such as word processors. Diary systems have not yet sold well enough to get the same attention and often face the additional problem of needing to be portable. However, recent developments such as the Z88 and Agenda Microwriter, although unable to replace the pocket diary, will replace some desk or company diaries. Once the market takes off, we may see faster evolution of such memory aids with spin-offs that are useful clinically.

Another possible route is to combine different technologies, in particular, using personal computer software which prints out pages for a portable diary. I tried this myself a few years ago, configuring a word-processing program to do the job. It worked very well for a while. I updated it as I made appointments, writing in by hand on the printout; every so often I entered the updates into the computer and printed out a new diary. As the novelty wore off, the intervals between putting the new entries into the computer increased, and eventually I found it a chore compared with a conventional diary to which I returned!

A much more sophisticated system called 'Portex' runs on the IBM PC and compatible personal computers and prints out pages in a variety of sizes and there is printed stationery available to go with it. Portex's own folders are a little smaller than Filofax, but Filofax size pages are available for it too. This will appeal to a limited number of people and represents an intermediate step on the route to portable, powerful and easy-to-use electronic diaries.

### Use with patients

Clearly using these sorts of aids to help patients with memory impairment presents many problems. I have already mentioned some of the most important ones, such as the difficulty of learning to use them and lack of portability. Some of the difficulties arise because even the better designed aids have not been designed specifically for people with clinical impairment. The cost can also be a problem.

However, in a minority of cases, a carefully selected aid could match the needs of a particular person. For example, a head-injured patient who used a personal computer for his or her work before the trauma could find one of the new personal organizer programs a useful aid in getting back to work, without being faced with the severe learning hurdle a computer-naïve patient would face.

A more readily available example is an approach taken by several clinical psychologists, including Rodger Wood (1983, personal communication), in which he successfully used an alarm watch combined with a conventional diary with two severely head-injured patients (PTAs of several months). Initially the alarms rang every 15 minutes to remind the patients to check their diaries for entries that had been written in for them. Although more conventional types of memory training had not been successful, this approach did help the patients and eventually they learned to check their diaries regularly and even to write in extra items.

This approach may be more appropriate in many cases than introducing the patient to unfamiliar technology; it's easier to remember how to use diaries. There is, for example, no screen to remember how to clear, a problem Barbara Wilson found with patients using the Memo Note 60. In many cases it may prove possible gradually to reduce the active reminders to a point at which the patients are left simply using normal diaries, aids that do not even mark them out as handicapped.

But like others this approach is only suitable in certain cases. Rodger Wood has noted some limitations. The patient must be able to write and to plan, and the staff doing the training must have the time and the motivation to do it regularly and frequently.

To finish with, it's worth noting that without spending any money at all, most of us could make far more effective use of active, specific and timely memory cues. Remember the skates left by the front door? They are likely to catch the child's attention at the time they need to be remembered and their specific significance is clear. While most of us are quite capable of devising such schemes, it is difficult to predict those occasions when we'll need an active reminder. So it is safer to develop a habit of assuming a reminder is necessary whenever there is a penalty attached to forgetting. I do try to use these methods myself, usually notes left in strategic places, but my frequent lapses are a constant source of amusement of my family, colleagues and friends, who gently remind me to practise what I preach!

## REFERENCES

Baddeley, A.D. (1982) *Your Memory: A User's Guide*, Macmillan, New York.

Black, P., Markowitz, R.S. and Cianci S. (1975) Recovery of motor function after lesions in motor cortex of monkey; in R. Porter and D.W. Fitzsimons (eds), *Outcome of Severe Damage to the Central Nervous System*. Ciba Foundation Symposium 34, Elsevier, Amsterdam.

Bower, G.H. and Clark, M.C. (1969) Narrative stories as mediators for serial learning, *Psychonomic Science*, **14**, 181–2.

Daniels P. (1988) *The Magic of Memory*, QED, BBC1 television broadcast, 6 February.

Davis, K.L., Mohs, R.C, Tinklenberg, J.R., Pfefferbaum, A., Hollister, L.E., and Kopell, B.S. (1978) Physostigmine: improvement of long-term memory processes in normal humans, *Science*, **201**, 272–4.

Ebbinghaus H.E. (1964) *Memory: A Contribution to Experimental Psychology* New York Dover (original work published 1885).

Ericsson, K.A., Chase, G.E. and Falcon, S. (1980) Acquisition of a memory skill, *Science*, **208**, 1181–2.

Gruneberg, M.M. (1987) *Linkword language courses in French, German, Spanish and Italian*, Corgi Books, London.

Harris, J.E. (1980) Memory aids people use: two interview studies, *Memory and Cognition*, **8**, 31–8.

Harris, J.E. (1984) Remembering to do things: a forgotten topic; in J.E. Harris and P.E. Morris (eds), *Everyday Memory, Actions and Absent-Mindedness*, Academic Press, London and Orlando.

Harris, J.E. and Sunderland, A. (1981) A brief survey of the management of memory disorders in rehabilitation units in Britain, *International Rehabilitation Medicine*, **3**, 206–9.

Harris, J.E. and Wilkins, A.J. (1982) Remembering to do things: a theoretical framework and an illustrative experiment, *Human Learning*, **1**, 123–36.

Higbee, K.L. (1977) *Your Memory: How it Works and How to Improve it*, Prentice Hall, Englewood-Cliffs, N.J.

Hunter, I.M.L. (1979) Memory in everyday life; in M.M. Gruneberg and P.E. Morris (eds), *Applied Problems in Memory*, Academic Press, London.

Kopelman, M.D. (1986) The cholinergic neurotransmitter system in human memory and dementia: a review, *Quarterly Journal of Experimental Psychology*, **38A**, 535–73.

Kreutzer, M.A., Leonard, C. and Flavell, J.H. (1975) An interview study of children's knowledge about memory, *Monographs of the Society for Research in Child Development*, **40** (1, Serial No. 159).

Landauer, T.K. and Bjork, R.A. (1978) Optimum rehearsal patterns and name learning; in M.M. Gruneberg, P.E. Morris and R.N. Sykes (eds.), *Practical Aspects of Memory*, Academic Press, London.

Lorayne, H. and Lucas, J. (1975) *The Memory Book*, W.H. Allen, London.

Masur, E.F., McIntyre, C.W. and Flavell, H.J. (1973) Developmental changes in the apportionment of study time in a multitrial free recall task, *Journal of Experimental Child Psychology*, **15**, 237–46.

Morris, P.E. (1977) Practical strategies for human learning and remembering; in M.J.A. Howe, *Adult Learning*, Wiley, Chichester and New York.

Moss, C. (1986) The watch that is ahead of its time, *Computer Guardian*, 21 August, 13.

Sitaram, N., Weingartner, H. and Gillin, J.C. (1978) Human serial learning: enhancement with arecoline and choline and impairment with scopolamine, *Science*, **201**, 274–6.

Wall, P.D. (1975) Signs of plasticity and reconnection in spinal cord damage; in R. Porter and D.W. Fitzsimons (eds), *Outcome of Severe Damage to the Central Nervous System*. Ciba Foundation Symposium 34, Elsevier, Amsterdam.

Wilson, B. and Moffat, N.J. (1984) Rehabilitation of memory for everyday life; in J.E. Harris and P.E. Morris (eds), *Everyday Memory, Actions and Absent-Mindedness*, Academic Press, London and Orlando.

Wood, R.Ll. (1983) Personal communication, 28 June.

Yates, F.A. (1966) *The Art of Memory*, Routledge and Kegan Paul, London.

# Chapter 4

# Strategies of memory therapy

## NICK MOFFAT

### INTRODUCTION

The previous chapter discussed methods of improving memory and provided a conceptual framework for their categorization. The present chapter examines these and other memory strategies in more detail, with particular reference to the rehabilitation of brain-injured people. It is emphasized that although a given memory strategy may be beneficial to one individual it may be of no value to another and indeed in some cases may actually prove to be detrimental. Varying responses to treatment will be largely dependent upon the nature and extent of a person's brain damage. As the process of selecting the most appropriate memory training strategies for a given individual will be described in the next chapter it will not be discussed further here.

In the first edition of this book, major strategies for memory therapy were described, including visual and verbal mnemonics. It was recognized that some of these strategies might be of limited value to amnesic people. It was also stated that there was little evidence for the effectiveness of simple memory exercises which relied upon the 'memory muscle' concept. Recent research has generally supported these earlier assertions. However, what has taken place in recent years has been an evaluation of certain memory strategies, such as the method of expanded retrieval and of vanishing cues which, together with clinical trials, suggest that these strategies can be used with a variety of patients and clinical problems. In addition, the value of external memory aids when tailored to suit individual needs, and the importance of systematic training in their use, has also been confirmed by recent studies. This chapter will describe these recent findings in more detail, and will also consider how other variables, including the reaction to having a memory loss, affect memory performance.

## VARIABLES WHICH MAY AFFECT MEMORY

The range of brain structures implicated in memory and the diversity of processes involved in remembering may explain why memory performance is readily disrupted by brain damage. However, memory performance and memory complaints may also be influenced by affective states (Kahn, Zarit, Hilbert and Niederehe, 1975) and by other cognitive variables, such as the speed of responding. Thus, the investigation of the inter-relationships between memory problems and other variables will be important because factors bearing upon amnesia may need to be dealt with before the true memory loss can be elucidated.

## REACTIONS TO THE ONSET OF MEMORY LOSS

The initial experience of brain damage may sensitize a patient, the family and possibly the staff to memory problems. Thus, in the case of people who have had a head injury there may be a period of retrograde (RA) and post-traumatic (PTA) amnesia surrounding the circumstances of the trauma, which in themselves may form a focus of concern.

Although PTA and some aspects of memory functioning may recover with time, it cannot be assumed that the patient's beliefs about memory performance, or those of others, are necessarily commensurate with the potential level of functioning. Thus, some head-injured patients may be concerned about their memory abilities, although this concern cannot be confirmed by memory tests. Feedback to these patients of their test results, and an explanation of the variety of types of memory, together with reassurance that only some severely head-injured patients suffer persistent memory problems, may help to reduce anxiety about memory performance, and encourage greater success in coping with everyday remembering.

The same principles can be applied to the non-confused elderly who may incorrectly attribute occasional absent-mindedness to age-related decline in memory abilities, or to the possibility of the early stages of dementia. This may result in a vicious circle of reported memory lapses, and anxiety or depression (resulting from the occurrence of these lapses), which in turn lead to further reported memory lapses. An outside factor which can add to this stress may occur when the person, or a relative, feels that memory performance would improve if the person tried harder. For example, we have recently been working with a woman who showed extreme anxiety (as measured by galvanic skin response as well as self-report) at the prospect of having to remember or to recall information. She has been taught to relax, and then remain relaxed, even while doing memory tasks. This has resulted in a marked improvement in her ability to cope with everyday memory tasks.

Stigsdotter and Backman (1989) have demonstrated that a multifactorial approach to memory therapy, which includes relaxation training, may be of particular benefit to elderly people. Their training consisted of recoding operations, attentional functions and relaxation which proved superior on the selective reminding test (both at post-training and at the six month follow-up) compared with the control condition, which consisted of training in problem-solving, logical thinking, and visuo-spatial skills.

Where there is an acute onset of memory loss the process of dealing with memory failures may be adversely affected by social factors. In the acute recovery stage the patient may have few demands placed upon him or her, with responsibilities involving remembering being carried out by others. There is a danger that this system of acute care may lag behind the progress of which the patient is capable. This may be an inadvertent process since the rate of recovery is not understood, or there may be maintaining factors which prolong the over-protection.

In order to delineate the psychological aspects of acute versus chronic care of amnesia, the operant model developed by Fordyce (1976) with regard to chronic pain will be used as a framework for exposition.

## OPERANT ANALYSIS OF FORGETTING BEHAVIOUR

The first question to be asked is whether forgetting behaviour is in fact being reinforced positively. A behavioural analysis of poor attention to task may reveal that a person receives staff attention for not working, or for alternative behaviours (e.g. asking what to do), but receives considerably less attention when working, since the staff then attend to other patients. The same analysis can be applied to the reinforcement that may occur for people with amnesia who repeatedly ask the same question. In order to overcome these problems it may be necessary to provide reinforcement for periods of time during which the person has not asked a repetitive question, or has attended to task; whilst systematically ignoring inappropriate behaviour. The time period required for attention to task, or not asking repetitive questions, can then be gradually increased as each stage in the therapy is achieved.

Indirect reinforcement of forgetting can occur if a person exaggerates symptoms in order to maximize a claim for compensation, although this is rarely seen in clinical practice. The same might apply when a person becomes over-dependent upon a memory aid. This is unlikely, since the problem usually involves getting amnesic patients to use or maintain the use of memory aids. Indirect reinforcement of forgetting may also occur when a patient avoids an unpleasant task by a convenient lapse of memory. Training to overcome this should aim to set tasks which are within the ability level of the patient, and the requirements should gradually be increased to correspond with and maximize progress.

It needs to be stated here, however, that a further question in operant analysis relates to reinforcement of appropriate remembering behaviour. Just as inappropriate behaviour may be reinforced so might appropriate behaviour be ignored. This might occur in a rest home or nursing home when an elderly person is not expected to use skills which are well-learned (e.g. cooking), or to remember to do things (e.g. shopping), since most of these tasks are performed by the staff. The non-reinforcement of remembering can also occur for amnesic people in other settings, since the person may be over-protected by family or staff. The fact that some severely amnesic people are not able to recall that they can do a particular task may mean that they do not attempt the task, unless this is deliberately encouraged by others. Also, some of the gradual forgetting of skills or information learned in therapy may be because of the lack of practice at these tasks at home.

In an attempt to increase the expectations of memory among nursing-home residents, Langer, Rodin, Beck, Weinman and Spitzer (1979) provided tokens for correctly answering questions which required the residents to find out information by the time of the next visit. The demands made upon the residents were gradually increased over time, and tokens exchanged for a gift at the end of the three-week period. It was found that the number of correct answers increased across the interviews, with the contingent token group supplying the correct information in a shorter period of time than those in the control conditions. Furthermore, there was generalization of improved memory to tests of immediate and remote memory among the contingent token group. The authors suggest that it might be worthwhile maintaining demands upon the memory of elderly people since, in the first part of their study, the no-treatment and minimal treatment groups showed a significant decline in memory over a six-week period, whilst the experimental group showed a significant increase in short-term memory.

In an earlier study (Langer and Rodin, 1976), elderly nursing home residents were given opportunities and encouraged to make their own decisions. As a result members of this group became more alert, happier and more active than the comparison group. Furthermore, eighteen months later those in the experimental group were found to have lived significantly longer than members of the comparison group (Rodin and Langer, 1977). Although there are some weaknesses in this study, the results are consistent with other evidence which suggests that maintaining the expectations of elderly people who are in particularly sheltered environments may help to maintain both the quality and the quantity of the remaining years.

Further evidence of the effects of increased emotional and intellectual stimulation amongst moderately demented patients in a nursing home comes from a study by Karlsson *et al.*, (1988). They found that although there was no change on psychological tests following two months of therapy, there were changes in the biochemistry of the cerebrospinal fluid (homovanillic acid) of these patients, but not amongst those who remained in a nursing home without this added stimulation.

For patients recovering from excessive alcohol consumption there is a suggestion that some aspects of recovery can be enhanced by practice at particular tasks (Goldman, 1987). However, there is very little evidence for the notion of a 'memory muscle' amongst amnesic subjects or controls. Thus, when memory training was used with alcoholics having memory problems, there was no benefit of this kind of practice compared with a control group (Godfrey and Knight, 1985). Even when densely amnesic patients have been taught to improve their recall of word lists (Kovner *et al*, 1983 and 1985), they may still remain disorientated for day and date. In one study, Korsakoff patients were taught to recall names of people and places within the hospital using rote rehearsal (Goldstein *et al.*, 1985; Goldstein and Malec, 1989). In keeping with the literature on reality orientation described later on in this chapter there was no evidence of the generalization of learning from one item to another.

These studies are in accordance with the majority of studies which have attempted to retrain or improve memory functioning by repeated practice. The results have been disappointing, both for normal subjects (Ericsson, Chase and Falcon, 1980; Herrmann, Buschke and Gall, 1987), and amnesic subjects (Milner, Corkin and Teuber, 1968; Brooks and Baddeley, 1976).

Therefore, there may be no support for such commonly used memory exercises as Kim's Game, which after all owes its origin to a story by Rudyard Kipling rather than being an experimentally validated technique. Memory is a complex process which is unlikely to respond as a 'mental muscle' (Harris and Sunderland, 1981). This is in keeping with the comments by Devor (1982), that 'the brain was designed to avoid injury, not to recover from it', and that the changes which occur 'are probably not designed to foster behavioural recovery of function . . . and in fact they may often be detrimental'.

As Gazzaniga (1978, p. 409) stated, 'in general, it is our belief that recovery almost invariably is the product of an alternative behavioural strategy being brought into play, with a patient in a sense, solving a behavioural task by taking a different "route to Rome"'. Therefore, for the therapist seeking ways of helping those with memory impairment, the strategies described below provide the most appropriate choice available, although there is considerable scope for innovation since memory therapy is still undergoing development and evaluation. As described below in more detail, improvements in performance are generally found to be very specific, and therefore training needs to be directly aimed at the problem the person with amnesia needs to master.

## ORGANIZATION OF MEMORY THERAPY

In order to devise a memory therapy programme it is necessary to assess the assets and deficits of the person, establish the priorities for therapy and then select the most appropriate training strategies. This is obviously an important and involved process, and further discussion will be confined to the selection and design of suitable training tasks, since the other considerations are dealt with elsewhere in this book, particularly in the next chapter.

There are a number of important ingredients which need to be included in the design of a rehabilitation programme.

### Selection of Task

The items chosen for training should be of practical concern to the person, and be considered worthwhile attainments. This is particularly important since there is very limited evidence of generalization from one task to another, and the training may take some time. As far as possible the task selected for training should include the impaired skill that one is trying to change, together with other skills which the subject can successfully demonstrate. The therapist should be able to vary the difficulty of the task from a level which would be simple for the patient to a level representing normal performance. At any given stage in therapy the difficulty level of the task should be set so that the number of errors made by the patient is kept to a minimum.

### Optimize learning

The difficulty of the task can be varied by altering the amount or complexity of information to be learned, the provision of learning strategies, the duration of retention expected, and the cues offered at the retrieval stage. Many of these features will be peculiar to the material or strategy being taught, but the general aim is to set the requirements at a level which ensures a reasonable degree of success. The precision teaching technique (Raybould and Solity, 1982) which has been applied in special education may prove to be particularly beneficial in aiding memory therapy continually to match the level of complexity of the task to the ability of the person. This method is particularly suitable for computer applications in memory therapy since the computer programme can be designed continually to adjust the duration of retention, or any other specified variable according to the level of performance over the preceding trials. The method of vanishing cues and the method of expanded retrieval, which are described in later sections, are particularly effective strategies for varying task difficulty and minimizing errors.

In addition, it is important to avoid the apparently common problem that amnesic people make of an early error being repeated thereafter. The errorless learning technique can be helpful in this respect since the task is given in such a way that the person is very likely to provide the correct answer.

### Evaluation

It is important to quantify the results and to provide feedback about performance, since progress in memory therapy may be slow at times and may require careful graphing in order to be noticed by the therapist or the patient. It may be valuable to provide standardized prompts if information to be learned is not freely recalled during training sessions, since this may reveal learning taking place before this is detected in measures of free recall (see later section on method of vanishing cues).

An additional consideration in the organization of memory therapy is the specification of the frequency and duration of training sessions, since it is generally preferable to have regular short training sessions rather than long training sessions.

## Maintenance

It is obviously difficult to determine the appropriate number of sessions before beginning memory therapy. Therefore, it may be more expedient to specify criteria to determine the termination of treatment. This will need to include lack of progress as well as the achievement of a specific aim. As mentioned earlier, progress may be slow and once achieved may not be maintained. It may therefore be worthwhile encouraging the person to over-learn a task in order to help maintain progress, and to provide regular follow-up booster sessions if necessary.

Having established some of the ways in which the therapist might organize the conditions for carrying out memory therapy, attention can be turned to memory strategies that the client could be taught in order to overcome specific memory complaints. The strategies outlined below are generally aimed at finding alternative means of remembering information, and may be considered to be ways of ameliorating a memory problem rather than restoring or retraining a memory deficit.

### EXTERNAL MEMORY AIDS

As Harris has described in the previous chapter, there is a good range of potential external memory aids. However, their incorporation in a memory programme may require careful planning. For example, although the Automatic Memorandum Clock (Shenton, 1975), which was available almost a century ago, possessed many of the requirements of a good cueing device, it proved a financial disaster!

The value of using a notebook compared with other more internal memory strategies was demonstrated by Zencius, Wesolowski and Burke (1990). The authors found that head injured subjects were more likely to be able to recall details of job adverts they had studied the day before if they had written the details in a memory notebook than if they had practised the items by verbal rehearsal, written rehearsal or acronym formation. From the results it appears that the training period was very short (two trials per condition) which may not have given sufficient time to test adequately the different strategies. Furthermore, this length of time did not provide evidence of the maintenance of any of the strategies, which would be important for establishing the practical benefits of the strategies for the individuals.

Obviously in order to be beneficial a memory aid must be fully utilized. The difficulty of proper use was demonstrated in a pilot project with a Korsakoff syndrome patient (Davies and Binks, 1983). The subject was given certain commands to remember, and other commands he wrote in a book. It was found that at the pre-arranged signal he had forgotten the significance of the signal and did not complete any of the actions. However, once he was prompted to use the book the written commands were obeyed, but not those previously committed to memory. This kind of system was successfully employed with a patient with early Alzheimer's disease who used a digital alarm watch which 'beeped' every hour to remind him to look at his daily programme and attend his appointments (Kurlychek, 1983). In the later section on reality orientation it is described how the mere provision of memory aids, such as sign-posts, may not be sufficient to ensure their use.

Relatives who are frequently answering questions or providing reassurance or instructions may be acting as external aids. As this can be irritating to the carers it may be possible to substitute written or recorded messages for verbal replies. For example, a woman with dementia had been getting out of bed and waking her sister about six times each night, although she would go back to bed when her sister asked her to. A tape recording of the sister telling her to go back to bed was made, and this tape loop was linked to a pressure mat beside the bed. The system was also linked to a timer so that the tape loop only operated between midnight and 6 a.m. After it had been installed, the sister was not disturbed at all between midnight and 6 a.m., except on one occasion when the mat moved and hence the lady was able to get out of bed without triggering the tape loop. She was still woken by her sister if they went to bed before midnight, and an additional written programme of activities was required to help the amnesic woman to remain occupied after she arose at 6 a.m. The sisters went away for a weekend, where they shared a room. Following this change of routine, the tape loop was no longer acceptable to the woman, and it had to be abandoned.

Bourgeois (1990) worked with three Alzheimer's disease patients and their spouses to produce a plastic wallet containing details covering three topics (my day, my life, and myself). The patients were trained to use these wallets in conversation, firstly with the experimenter and then with their spouse. All of the patients made significantly more statements of fact, and fewer ambiguous utterances after training, which was maintained at the three- and six-week follow up.

External memory aids may not only be valuable for the memory-impaired person, but may also prove a suitable aide memoire for carers. Thus, in the Davies and Binks study a prompt card was designed to be shown to others so that they interacted appropriately with Mr F., the amnesic person. The prompt card provided specific guidelines which enabled the subject to note important dates and addresses and check them. Mr F was also given role play training in how to ask someone to jot something down in his book. In this way the use of the aid became fully established in his daily routine, and was still in use at a one-year follow up.

As can be seen from the above, some patients with dementia or severe amnesia can learn to use external memory aids. The next section will outline how patients can learn to recall information, or make best use of external memory aids by following the principles of reality orientation.

REALITY ORIENTATION

The original goal of reality orientation (RO) was to meet the sensory and emotional needs of long-stay patients by encouraging nursing assistants to spend more time in one-to-one personal contact with patients, to provide stimulating activities for patients, and to encourage certain staff attitudes (Folsom, 1968).

The main guidelines for RO were summarized by Hanley (1986) as follows.

1. Presentation of new information in a variety of formats including routine communication and special learning groups
2. Correction of confused behaviour
3. Prompting, rehearsal and reinforcement of adaptive behaviour
4. Provision of memory aids as prostheses for memory problems.

The emphasis has gradually changed so that most of the RO studies have been concerned with helping the elderly confused patient, particularly with regard to cognitive and behavioural functioning. However, it has been applied with other people, such as those who have suffered a head injury (Cerny and McNeny, 1983); and Corrigan *et al.*, 1985). Most studies have involved in-patients, but there have been a growing number of accounts of RO with day patients (e.g. Greene *et al.*, 1983). In addition, some authors have discussed the possibility of using RO with family members (e.g. Hanley, 1986; Moffat, 1989).

The two main ways in which RO has been carried out have been informal RO (also known as '24-hour RO'), and formal RO (also known as 'RO groups' or 'classroom RO').

The basic format of reality orientation, whether 24-hour or classroom sessions, includes reminding patients who they are, who is speaking to them, providing information about time and place, and giving a commentary about what is going on. It is suggested that the therapist speaks clearly, keeping statements specific and brief. The patient is encouraged to rehearse the information provided and to converse with the staff and patients. The staff member requires some knowledge of the patient's family and personal history, since it is important to verify information provided by the patient. References by the patient to the past should be responded to accordingly (for example, 'Yes, you used to live in Basingstoke').

Formal RO sessions have been described as a supplement to informal RO by some authors (Drummond *et al*, 1978), although they have been used on their own in some studies. A review of these formal sessions is provided in Chapter 9, and so will not be described further.

The two main studies of informal RO (Zepelin, Wolffe and Kleinplatz, 1981, and Davis, 1984) did not show any short- or long-term benefits of informal RO alone, although both studies found some benefit of combining formal sessions with the informal RO.

The studies mentioned above may have suffered from the same problems reported by Hanley (1981a) cited in Hanley (1984). He observed that training staff in RO did not produce any changes in either the number of inter-actions staff had with patients, or in the mean number of RO behaviours present per interaction. This was in spite of the staff believing that they were carrying out these procedures.

If the problem is that staff do not initiate RO behaviour, then the modified informal RO approach included in the study by Reeve and Ivison (1985) may be more acceptable. The aim was for the staff to respond to residents' initia-tives rather than to initiate the interactions themselves. This resulted in improvements in cognitive and behavioural functioning which were maintained for twelve weeks. A limitation in the interpretation of this study is that the effects of this modified informal RO procedure cannot be separated from the environmental manipulations which were also carried out, such as the addition of signposts and colour coding of doors. As outlined in the next sec-tion, these may be significant treatment variables in their own right.

An alternative to concentrating on verbal information is to teach patients to find their own way around the ward environment by putting up appropriate signs and then using these signs in practice at route finding within the ward. The addition of signposts to the ward has produced improvements in orientation in one study (Gilleard, Mitchell and Riordin, 1981), but not in two other studies (Hanley, 1981b, and McCartney, 1984). A more consistent improvement in specific route finding has been found when patients have been actively taught to use the signs (Gilleard *et al.*, 1981; Hanley, 1981b; Hanley, McGuire and Boyd, 1981; and, to some extent, McCartney, 1984).

Hanley (1986) provided further evidence of the importance of training people with dementia in the use of external memory aids. He found that a confused elderly person was only able to use a diary to keep appointments and recall orientation items which had been written in it, following specific training to do so; and this ability relapsed once the specific training had ceased. It may be that an active reminder is required to ensure maintenance, such as the combined use of an alarm watch and a daily programme for a person with early Alzheimer's disease to check what to do every hour (Kurlychek, 1983).

One of the features of the work on ward orientation training has been a concern with problems of direct relevance to the person, such as finding the way around the ward (e.g. Hanley, 1981b); knowing what to do at certain times of day (Kurlychek, 1983); and how to find things in the house (Moffat, 1984a). Environmental alterations may prove worthwhile with some confused elderly people, particularly where there is active training in the use of these prosthetic environments.

In general the studies of RO do not provide support for the informal approach, mainly because staff do not incorporate RO-based statements in their interactions (Hanley, 1981a). Part of the difficulty arises from the lack of specificity as to what staff should do, since over-zealous use of RO might be seen as unacceptable to the patient. Furthermore, traditional informal RO does not provide specific reinforcement for appropriate staff behaviour.

A more structured approach to RO does appear to result in specific gains. Thus, ward orientation training may help with learning specific routes around the ward. Furthermore, the formal approach to RO, whether in groups or individually, does appear to improve orientation for those items which have been taught (see Wilson and Moffat, this volume).

The multiplicity of problems which can occur amongst those with dementia means that it is important to take into account the person's neuropsychological assets and deficits, as well as the person's environment and social interactions (Hodge, 1984). For example, a behavioural programme for incontinence needs to determine whether the person can find the way to the toilet; training to reduce wandering needs to determine the effects of lighting in aiding orientation (Cameron, 1941); and the treatment of repetitive themes needs to determine whether there is an inability to remember the answer to the repetitive question (Wilson, 1984), or whether the behaviour has been maintained by the attention of others (Goldstein and Ruthven, 1983; Moffat, 1984b). Considerable expertise is required in order to set up a programme, and the success of a programme will also depend upon the support of all those involved. This is perhaps why so few studies have evaluated behavioural approaches with confused elderly people and why RO should not be considered an 'off the peg' treatment (Hanley, 1986).

Although a number of authors have written about involving relatives in the use of RO, this may need to be conducted carefully. Zarit, Zarit and Reever (1982) found that involving relatives in memory groups for their confused dependant resulted in the relatives becoming more depressed. This may have been because they then realized the extent of the person's problems. However, as stressed earlier, perhaps suitable training programmes can be devised (e.g. treatment of repetitive themes), which will be of benefit to both the confused elderly and the family. This will be of considerable importance, since the majority of the confused elderly are presumed to be living in the community, and caring can result in considerable strain for these relatives.

This section has outlined the potential of RO for teaching particular items of orientation to severely amnesic patients. The next section will outline various mnemonic strategies which can be used to overcome some of the problems which people with memory problems frequently complain about, such as difficulty recalling the names of people.

## VISUAL IMAGERY

The memory strategies described below make use of the formation of a mental picture of information to aid remembering.

## MEMORY FOR NAMES

The face-name association method involves transforming the person's name (e.g. Angela Webster) into a mental image (e.g. in this case involving an angel, a web and a star). Secondly, a distinctive feature of the person is then linked to the mental image. For example, if the distinctive feature of Angela Webster is her hair, the image might be of an angel and a star caught in a web, made out of her hair. The advantage of this system is that it provides a unique link between the person's name and face, which is in keeping with the finding that the images should be interacting but need not be bizarre (Wollen, Weber and Lowry, 1972).

In order for this procedure to be effective with memory impaired people it may be necessary to provide the mental image for the person, perhaps as a drawing. It appears that the simpler the method of constructing the mental image the better: whilst the more elaborate face-name association technique may be possible for normal subjects (McCarty, 1980), it appears to be impractical for many brain-damaged individuals (Glasgow *et al.*, 1977; and Wilson, 1981). However, it appears that the small number of names taught to brain-injured people and the way in which practice can be spaced out by using the multiple baseline design (Hersen and Barlow, 1976) may reduce any confusion between the names to be learned and the respective faces.

Using the simplified visual imagery method described above, amnesic patients have been able to recall significantly more names following visual imagery than rote rehearsal practice (Moffat, 1984b; Wilson, 1981 and 1987). Furthermore, in the study mentioned in Moffat (1984b), one of the two head injured subjects continued to recall more names following visual imagery than rote rehearsal at the one-, three- and six-month follow ups.

## Peg-type mnemonics

In the first edition of this book a range of other visual mnemonics were described. These were mainly peg-type mnemonics, which involve the learning of a set of standard peg words to which are associated further items to be remembered. The three main variants of the peg mnemonic are the rhyming peg method; the phonetic system (sometimes also referred to as the hook or digit-sound method) and the method of loci. It was stated in the first edition that these mnemonics were of limited practical benefit to people, particularly anyone with a severe memory problem. This is partly because of the difficulty in learning the peg system before it can be applied. Also the peg type mnemonics are generally suitable for lists of words (e.g. shopping lists) which can be written down and recalled using external memory aids without the necessity of using elaborate mnemonics. Thus, even some of the authors of memory enhancement books, such as Cermak (1980) have found few personal benefits from visual imagery. However, as has been described with regard to visual imagery for names, in some circumstances visual imagery mnemonics may be able to provide worthwhile and long-lasting gains for patients with generalized brain damage.

Discussion will now turn to verbal mnemonics which have undergone some investigation with clinical populations.

### VERBAL STRATEGIES

A number of variables have been found to influence the amount of verbal information recalled by either normal or amnesic subjects. These have included organizing of words in categories according to their meaning or sound (Baddeley and Warrington, 1973).

Alternatively, learning pairs of words (such as clock-glove) has been facilitated by the addition of verbal links such as hand (clock-hand-glove). This has resulted in fewer trials being required to learn the word pairs (Cermak, 1976).

A further strategy involves forming a story linking items to be remembered (Gianutsos and Gianutsos, 1979). This task has proved difficult for some amnesic people (Crovitz,

Harvey and Horn, 1979) and in many respects can be considered a visual imagery procedure since the linking of each item in the list with the next may be achieved using a visual image.

In general, these mnemonics are only applicable to experimental tasks, and would be inappropriate for dealing with everyday problems.

### Study method

A common difficulty for people with memory problems is remembering written prose such as newspaper articles. Various techniques have been proposed to help study this type of material, using a series of stages.

Glasgow *et al.*, (1977) used the following steps to assist the verbal memory disorder of a young severely head-injured woman.

Preview:   Establish the general order of the text.
Question:  Think of the main questions about the material.
Read:      Read the text carefully.
State:     Repeat the information that has been read.
Test:      Check that the text has been understood and the questions which were posed were satisfactorily answered.

Using selected passages the PQRST method resulted in superior recall compared with a rehearsal condition and the subject's own pre-intervention strategy. However, part of the benefit of the PQRST method was presumably derived from the extra time taken to apply the PQRST method. During the second phase of the study the PQRST training successfully generalized to the remembering of newspaper articles.

Wilson (1987) has carried out a series of studies of the PQRST technique with people with memory problems. In general, the PQRST strategy was superior to a rehearsal condition, particularly for recall after a delay interval. However, the more severely amnesic patients were unable to recall information without prompts at the delay interval, whereas the mildly amnesic patients were able freely to recall information at the immediate and delayed recall attempts. These studies were conducted using newspaper articles or short passages. The method can also be applied with daily activities such as watching the television news or television programmes, particulary if prepared worksheets are kept near the television. A bookmark with the details of the study method written on it may help with the maintenance and generalization of this skill in everyday life. It may be important to teach each of the stages of this strategy, so that, for example, patients have learned how to identify the key points of a story before they are expected to recall them after a delay interval.

### Method of vanishing cues

This strategy involves practice at remembering something (e.g. a person's name), followed by attempts at recall using prompts which are gradually increased until recall is achieved. For example, if the name 'Sam' is to be remembered then at recall the prompts would be:

| Order of presentation | Prompts | Number of prompts |
|---|---|---|
| First | – – – | 0 |
| Second | S – – | 1 |
| Third | S A – | 2 |
| Fourth | S A M | 3 |

For each practice trial the number of prompts are recorded, with evidence of learning being denoted by a reduction in the number of prompts required for recall. This measure can also be used to determine the carry-over of learning from one training session to another.

The method is based on two well-established and related principles. First, the behavioural technique of providing prompts which are graded in degree of assistance (e.g. verbal, gestural and then physical) in order to facilitate learning. Second, the facilitation of performance amongst controls and people with memory problems on tasks such as word-fragment completion and word identification (Warrington and Weiskrantz, 1974). To date, the main applications of this method have been with verbal information, but it could be evaluated with non-verbal tasks, if suitable graded prompts can be devised.

The main research which has described and evaluated the method of vanishing cues has been carried out at the Unit for Memory Disorders in Toronto by Glisky and Schacter. They found that memory-impaired patients could learn a small computer vocabulary which was retained for six weeks (Glisky, Schacter and Tulving, 1986a). Their second study showed that head-injured patients could learn to write and edit simple programs, and use some disk storage and retrieval operations, with retention of this learning being observed over one month (Glisky, Schacter and Tulving, 1986b).

In a further study they demonstrated that amnesic patients with various etiologies could learn how to operate a computer, and that the knowledge and skills acquired could be retained for up to nine months. The good retention of this knowledge over time was helped by the significant amount of over-learning in the first place (Glisky and Schacter, 1988).

One of the subjects in the study mentioned above had been able to cope with a simple clerical job. However, this job was going to be phased out, and so she was successfully trained to carry out a complex computer data entry task in the laboratory, and with additional training and guidance in the work-place she was able to perform the task as accurately and quickly as experienced data-entry employees. She was able to remain in this part-time employment for at least six months (Glisky and Schacter, 1987). She had great difficulty with the task at first, and her learning was always slow. Despite her level of amnesia and low verbal intelligence (79) following her herpes simplex encephalitis, she had two assets which helped her. These were her ability to persevere at a task, and to monitor her responses. The fact that the task was very specific, and did not require problem-solving also helped her, since the learning was very specific. Thus, she could not recall details of her job, and did not show any improvements on other cognitive tasks.

The work of Glisky and Schacter has not been widely applied by others so far. However, the present author has

used this strategy over the last six years, and has demonstrated that it can be widely applied as long as certain
considerations are taken into account.

The range of potential applications of the method of
vanishing cues is large. For example, it can be used to
overcome naming difficulties, and in the relearning or new
learning of basic items of orientation with patients with
dementia. It can also be used to teach spatial tasks; writing
ability following dysgraphia; and in motor tasks such as
drinking from a cup, or positioning a wheelchair (see also
Wilson, and Wood, this volume). The main requirement is
the construction of a graded series of prompts which can be
introduced systematically.

The procedure need not be administered by computer, as
Glisky and Schacter had used in their work. Booklets, or a
framework with a slider which is pulled, can be used to reveal
the letters one-by-one. In this way some patients can learn
to use the system at home on their own, or with guidance
by a family member. Some families have gone on to use the
booklets to teach information which had not been set up by
the author.

A modification which has been incorporated into some of
the training has been the withholding of the first letter of
the to-be-recalled word until last (i.e. providing the second,
and then subsequent letters, and then finally including the
first letter of the word). This was done for several reasons.
First, patients may be able to recall spontaneously the first
letter of the word. Second, the provision of the first letter
is a disproportionately effective retrieval cue. Third, there
was some suggestion (Glisky, 1985) that patients became
dependent upon the provision of this first letter prompt
for recall.

The method of vanishing cues can be a powerful strategy in
memory therapy. A limitation of the strategy is that it does not
have a clear rationale regarding the frequency of practice trials
within a session, or the length of time between sessions. This
can be overcome by combining the method of vanishing cues
with the method of expanded retrieval, in order to provide a
comprehensive rehabilitation programme.

## EXPANDED RETRIEVAL PRACTICE

Expanded retrieval practice is based on experimental evidence suggesting that the longer the distracting interval from the first to the second successful recall attempt, the greater the likelihood of recall at a third recall attempt (Bjork, 1988). It is suggested that the optimal rehearsal pattern involves testing an item after a short retention interval and then, if recall is successful, gradually to increase the duration of each subsequent retention interval, hence forming a series with expanding retention intervals in between tests of recall.

The method of expanded retrieval practice can be applied within a training session by increasing the time interval (Schacter, Rich and Stampp, 1985) or the number of intervening items (Landauer and Bjork, 1978) between practice trials. It can also be used across days by increasing the number of intervening days between retrieval attempts (e.g. 2, 4, 8, 14, 22, 32, 44, 58, 74, 92 and 112 days since the last test) as used by Linton (1988) when learning plant names.

Expanded retrieval practice has been applied in educational settings (Rea and Modigliani, 1988). However, despite suggestions that the technique could be applied to brain-damaged subjects (Moffat, 1984b), only one experimental study (Schacter, Rich and Stampp, 1985), and one applied study (Moffat, 1989) have been published.

The author has used the method of expanded retrieval in the rehabilitation of a range of clinical problems, including retraining of letter writing (dysgraphia); naming ability; and relearning or new learning of items of general knowledge and also of verbal orientation. There appears to be no reason why the method needs to be confined to verbal skills, and hence it could be used to practise motor or other skills.

The method has been applied with subjects who have very different degrees of memory impairment. As expected, in a study of patients with dementia, over an eleven-week period, there was a significant relationship between the number of items of verbal orientation learned during this time and the level of cognitive impairment ($r=0.95$, $p<0.05$).

The method of delivery of the procedure has also varied according to the ability level, and circumstances of the patient. For the most able patients the procedure has been self-administered, using prepared booklets or instruction sheets. A kitchen timer has been used as an active reminder of the end of the required retention interval, and as a cue for recall of a written question. The booklets have also been used in a diary format to provide practice of items on an expanding retrieval basis across days, covering at least a month.

The procedure has been used in one-to-one training sessions carried out by a therapist or a family member with the patient. Training sessions have also been presented on a computer, which varies the next retention interval according to the performance on the preceding recall attempt. Five different items of information can be run independently, but concurrently, using this program. Various distraction tasks can be presented by the program during the time interval in between recall attempts.

A further computer program was written which held the question and answer to specific items of orientation, and acted as a reminder for staff working in a day hospital with patients who had dementia. At appropriate time intervals (see computer program described above) an audible alarm sounded to remind staff to look at the computer screen and then work with the particular patient on a specific item of orientation. The computer program also dealt with all data recording and analysis, which added to the acceptability by staff of this form of expanded retrieval practice.

A number of considerations need to be borne in mind when designing a therapy program incorporating expanded retrieval practice.

### The schedule of expanded retrieval practice

A simple rule is to double the time interval for each successive retention interval (e.g. 0, 2, 4, 8, 16 and then approximately 30 minutes, followed by 1, 2 and then 4 hours) in between retrieval attempts. The same rule of doubling can be applied across successive days if retrieval attempts are planned that far in advance.

The expanding series needs to be modified to suit individual patients, and the wide variations in performance of the same patient when learning even apparently similar types of information. For example in the study with dementia patients, the retention interval was only increased when an item had been successfully recalled on three consecutive trials at a particular retention interval.

A model is being developed which will help to determine the most appropriate expansion intervals for an individual. This model can take into account the effect that recall on a preceding trial has on the probability of recall on a subsequent trial. This is an improvement on the existing probability model (Bjork, 1988) which is not applicable to the expanding series used in current applied studies.

## Criteria if failure occurs

The available evidence, and detailed analysis of the performance of individual patients reveal that once a patient fails to recall at a particular retention interval, then performance on the next retention interval is severely impaired. This decrement in future performance is noted even if there have been further successful recall trials at this retention interval. Therefore, failure to recall should be avoided if at all possible. One way of reducing the problem is to provide cues to recall (see method of vanishing cues) so that at least partial success can be achieved. This method was incorporated into the study of dementia patients so that morale and performance levels remained high.

Failure to recall an item need not result in a shortening of the next retention interval, since further trials at the same retention interval may sometimes prove satisfactory. However, failure may also indicate fatigue and indicate that the therapy session has already been too long.

## Length of therapy session

With more able patients, who progress through an expanding retrieval series, only the first half-hour of training requires regular and concentrated effort. Thereafter the time commitment decreases over the course of the day, as outlined below.

| Time interval in between recall attempts | Time to test recall |
|---|---|
| Initial practice | 10.00 a.m. |
| 0 minutes | 10.00  " |
| 2  " | 10.02  " |
| 4  " | 10.06  " |
| 8  " | 10.15  "  (approx.) |
| 16  " | 10.30  "      " |
| 30  "  (approx.) | 11.00  " |
| 1 hour | 12.00 |
| 2 hours | 2.00 p.m. |
| 4  " | 6.00  " |
| Next day | Next day |

However, with patients who have a more cautious expansion series, or who fail during the practice trials, a pre-determined maximum duration for a session needs to be established. For patients with dementia, a half-hour session can be planned for the morning, and then again for the afternoon.

### Training plan and evaluation

In general it is preferable to learn one item at a time, and then add a further item once this has been learned to a set criterion. Thus, for one woman who had memory loss following anoxia, 73 items of general knowledge was learned over a three-month period, with one item being practised virtually every day. She was able to recall 68% of the items at one week, and 54% at an average of three and a half weeks following training of each item. Even in this example a careful monitoring of success on different retention intervals was carried out to reduce redundant retention intervals, and maintain high levels of performance during training.

There is a need for further refinement of expanded retrieval procedures with people with memory problems, and also for controlled trials of expanded retrieval versus matched fixed interval schedules. However, the method does have considerable potential since it can be applied to a range of practical problems and requires little cognitive effort from the patient.

## PROCEDURAL MEMORY

In recent years there has been increasing interest in studying the type of task that people with amnesia can remember. One area that has been studied is that of learning to perform actions. This has been called motor memory, subject-performed tasks, and also procedural memory. The range of tasks studied includes learning to do mirror-star drawing, pursuit-rotor, and bi-manual tracking (Corkin, 1968); as well as learning to do the Tower of Hanoi Puzzle in as few moves as possible (Cohen, 1984); and remembering instructions, either those carried out by the subject or by the experimenter (Cohen and Heath, 1988).

Some of the earlier studies demonstrated that amnesic subjects showed normal performance on a range of these procedural tasks, but were impaired on tests of declarative (e.g. recall and recognition) memory (Brooks and Baddeley, 1976; Cohen, 1984; Cohen and Squire, 1980). This meant that some of the subjects could do the task, but not recall having done it, and could not recognize items from the procedural task.

There has been some suggestion that declarative memory is dependent on the diencephalic medial temporal lobe system (Squire and Cohen, 1984), and hence is impaired in, for example, patients with alcoholic Korsakoff's syndrome. Furthermore, it has been proposed that the basal ganglia may be important for procedural skills (e.g. Martone *et al.*, 1984) and hence may be impaired in patients with Parkinson's disease, and some patients with Huntington's disease.

In support of this distinction between declarative and procedural memory some studies have found a double dissociation in that Huntington's disease patients show performance deficits on procedural but not declarative tasks, whilst amnesic patients show the opposite pattern of effects (Heindel, Butters and Salmon, 1988; Martone *et al.*, 1984).

Unfortunately, in more recent studies the evidence has been less clear-cut, resulting in the need to add various provisos. First, there can be dissociations between tasks considered to be procedural, and therefore they must differ in some component processes (Harrington *et al.*, 1990).

Second, the more the task resembles ordinary everyday skills, the more it is likely to involve both procedural and declarative processes (Kendrick, Healey and Brown, 1988). Third, not all amnesic people can acquire cognitive skills normally, and therefore this type of learning must depend upon the nature of the neuroanatomic system (Butters *et al.*, 1985).

It can be seen from all this that procedural learning is difficult to define since it seems to refer *post hoc* to any motor, perceptual, or cognitive skills amnesics learn and remember in normal fashion' (Beatty *et al.*, 1987).

In general it appears that amnesic patients (with the exception of some patients with Parkinson's or Huntington's disease) may be able to acquire and perform certain procedural tasks. These tasks may be of value to the person in gaining employment (such as routine assembly or data-entry jobs); or in leisure pursuits such as bowls or golf. The problem is that the preserved learning may only be useful for part of the required skills so that for example two amnesic patients the author is working with are able to go on improving their handicap at golf, but they have to rely on external memory aids to keep count of the number of strokes at each hole, and to record their performance. In addition, they both have problems with the names of the people with whom they regularly play golf, and with the declarative memory involved in conversations on the golf course.

The fact that amnesic patients can learn procedural skills may help with maintaining morale, since it offers specific avenues for training, and some optimism for future progress.

An advantage of procedural learning is that tasks can be learned directly, and hence do not have to rely upon elaborate mnemonics. Therefore, the person could go on to learn new skills with appropriate guidance. However, it has to be recognized that the person may need encouragement and augmented freedback of performance for subsequent recall of the performed act.

Although the available evidence has concentrated on simple tasks, it may be that more varied problem-solving can be taught, since some amnesic subjects have been able to learn the look-ahead puzzle of the Tower of Hanoi (Cohen, 1984).

It would seem that procedural memory probably offers the greatest potential in the next few years for the development of memory rehabilitation.

Some people with memory problems do not recognize the extent of their amnesia. Exercises to improve metacognition can be devised which provide feedback about the direction and magnitude of the difference between estimated and actual performance on a variety of tasks. This can be carried out in individual or group therapy (see Wilson and Moffat, this volume), and in microcomputer-based practice (Vroman, Kellar and Cohen, 1989).

In addition, some patients do not recall or utilize strategies which they have learned which might improve their memory performance. This has been recognized as a problem amongst people who have learning difficulties, as well as those who have a brain injury. Teaching subjects to use executive strategies in order to become more self-sufficient has been tried for some years with people with learning difficulties (Brown, 1978), but has only recently been tried systematically with those who have had a head injury (Lawson and Rice, 1989). These authors trained a young head-injured male to follow an acronym (WSTC) which asked him to check:

What are you asked to do?
Select a strategy for the task
Try out a strategy
Check out how the strategy was working.

The strategies were initially aimed at improving his test-taking performance (e.g. list learning, paired associate and spatial imagery strategy training) and were only later applied to his direct educational needs (e.g. place names in geography, remembering details of stories in English). The results do indicate some improvements in test performance immediately following training, and at a six-month follow up. However, the benefits appear to be very specific, since there was no improvement in the reading comprehension test, and he did not maintain use of his diary.

Foxx, Marchand-Martella, Martella *et al.* (1988) taught

head-injured adults everyday problem-solving skills in the following four main areas:

Community awareness and transportation
Medication, alcohol and drugs
Stating one's rights
Emergencies, injuries and safety.

There was evidence of a treatment effect since the treated subjects improved in all areas. This was maintained across non-cued conditions, and there was some generalization, whereas there was little or no change in the control group over the same period.

Further and more systematic evaluation of the executive strategies is warranted because of the frequent difficulty of helping patients to generalize and maintain the use of memory strategies. It is also a challenge for the therapist to find strategies which are as useful to the patient as possible, and which minimize the difficulty that many have found in finding a practical application for a well-established strategy which has been investigated only with experimental tasks.

## REFERENCES

Baddeley, A.D. and Warrington, E.K. (1973) Memory coding and amnesia, *Neuropsychologia*, **11**, 159–65.

Beatty, W., Salmon, D., Bernstein, N., *et al.* (1987) Procedural learning in a patient with amnesia due to hypoxia, *Brain and Cognition*, **6**, 386–402.

Bjork, R.A. (1988) Retrieval practice and the maintenance of knowledge in M.M. Gruneberg P.E. Morris and R.N. Sykes (eds), *Practical Aspects of Memory: current research and issues*, J. Wiley and Sons, Chichester, 283–8.

Bourgeois, M. (1990) Enhancing conversation skills in patients with Alzheimer's disease using a prosthetic memory aid, *Journal of Applied Behaviour Analysis*, **23**, 29–42.

Brooks, D.N. and Baddeley, A.D. (1976) What can amnesics learn? *Neuropsychologia*, **14**, 111–22.

Brown, A.L. (1978) Knowing when, where and how to remember: a problem in metacognition; in R. Glasser (ed), *Advances in Instructional Psychology*, Lawrence Erlbaum Associates, Hillsdale, New Jersey.

Butters, N., Wolfe, J., Martone, M., Granholm, E. and Cermak, L. (1985) Memory disorders associated with Huntington's disease: verbal recall, verbal recognition and procedural learning, *Neuropsychologia*, **23**, 729–43.

Cameron, D.E. (1941) Studies in senile nocturnal delirium, *Psychiatric Quarterly*, **15**, 47–53.

Cermak, L.S. (1976) The encoding capacity of a patient with amnesia due to encephalitis, *Neuropsychologia*, **14**, 311–26.

Cermak, L.S. (1980) Comments on imagery as a therapeutic mnemonic: in L.W. Poon, J.L. Fozard, L.S. Cermak, D. Arenberg, and L.W. Thompson (eds), *New Directions in Memory and Aging*, Lawrence Erlbaum Associates, Hillsdale, New Jersey.

Cerny, J. and McNeny, R. (1983) Reality orientation therapy: in M. Rosenthal. E.R. Griffith, M.R. Bond, and J.D. Miller (eds), *Rehabilitation of the Head Injured Adult*, F.A. Davis & Co., Philadelphia.

Cohen, N. (1984) Preserved learning capacity in amnesia: evidence for multiple memory systems; in L.R. Squire and N. Butters (eds), *Neuropsychology of Memory*, Guildford Press, New York.

Cohen, N. and Squire, L.R. (1980) Preserved learning and retention of pattern analysing skills and dissociations of knowing how and knowing that, *Science*, **210**, 207–10.

Cohen, R. and Heath, M. (1988) Recall probabilities for enacted instructions; in M.M. Gruneberg, P.E. Morris and R.N. Sykes (eds), *Practical Aspects of Memory*, Volume 1, 421–6, J. Wiley & Sons, Chichester.

Corkin, S. (1968) Acquisition of motor skill after bilateral medial temporal-lobe excision, *Neuropsychologia*, **6**, 255–64.

Corrigan, J.D., Arnett, J.A., Houck, L.J. and Jackson, R.D. (1985) Reality orientation for brain injured patients: group treatment and monitoring of recovery, *Archives of Physical Medicine and Rehabilitation*, **66**, 626–30.

Crovitz, H., Harvey, M. and Horn, R. (1979) Problems in the acquisition of imagery mnemonics: three brain damaged cases, *Cortex*, **15**, 225–34.

Davies, A.D.M. and Binks, M.G. (1983) Supporting the residual memory of a Korsakoff patient, *Behavioural Psychotherapy*, **11**, 62–74.

Davis, J. (1984) *Reality orientation therapy: a study to investigate some treatment outcome variables in patients and nursing staff*, Dissertation for the Diploma in Clinical Psychology, British Psychological Society, Leicester.

Devor, M. (1982) Plasticity in the adult nervous system; in L.S. Illis, E.M. Sedgwick and H.T. Glanville (eds), *Rehabilitation of the Neurological Patient*, Blackwell Scientific Publications, Oxford.

Drummond, L., Kirchoff, L. and Scarborough, D.R. (1978) A practical guide to reality orientation: a treatment approach for confusion and disorientation, *Gerontologist*, **18**, 568–73.

Ericsson, K.A., Chase, W.G. and Falcon, S. (1980) Acquisition of a memory skill, *Science*, **208**, 1181–2

Folsom, J.C. (1968) Reality orientation for the elderly mental patient, *Journal of Geriatric Psychiatry*, **1**, 291–307.

Fordyce, W.E. (1976) *Behavioral Methods for Chronic Pain and Illness*, Mosby, St Louis.

Foxx, R., Marchand-Martella, N., Martella, R., Braunling-McMorrow, D. and McMorrow, M. (1988) Teaching a problem-solving strategy to closed head-injured adults, *Behavioral Residential Treatment*, **3**, 193–210.

Gazzaniga, M.S. (1978) Is seeing believing: notes on clinical recovery; in S. Finger (ed), *Recovery from Brain Damage*, Plenum Press, New York. 409–14.

Gianutsos, R. and Gianutsos, J. (1979) Rehabilitating the verbal recall of brain injured patients by mnemonic training: an experimental demonstration using single case methodology, *Journal of Clinical Neuropsychology*, **1**, 117–35.

Gilleard, C., Mitchell, R.G. and Riordin, J. (1981) Ward orientation training with psychogeriatric patients, *Journal of Psychiatry*, **131**, 90–4.

Glasgow, R.E., Zeiss, R.A., Barrera, M. and Lewinsohn, P.M. (1977) Case studies on remediating memory deficits in brain damaged individuals, *Journal of Clinical Psychology*, **33**, 1049–54.

Glisky, E. (1985) Personal communication.

Glisky, E. and Schacter, D. (1987) Acquisition of domain-specific knowledge in organic amnesia: training for computer-related work, *Neuropsychologia*, **25**, 893–906.

Glisky, E. and Schacter, D. (1988) Long-term retention of computer learning by patients with memory disorders. *Neuropsychologia*, **26**, 173–8.

Glisky, E., Schacter, D. and Tulving, E. (1986a) Learning and retention of computer-related vocabulary in amnesic patients: method of vanishing cues, *Journal of Clinical and Experimental Neuropsychology*, **8**, 292–312.

Glisky, E., Schacter, D. and Tulving, E. (1986b) Computer learning by memory-impaired patients: acquisition and retention of complex knowledge, *Neuropsychologia*, **24**, 313–28.

Godfrey, H.P.D. and Knight, R.G. (1985) Cognitive rehabilitation and memory functioning in amnesiac alcoholics, *Journal of Consulting and Clinical Psychology*, **53**, 555–7.

Goldman, M.S. (1987) The role of time and practice in recovery of function of alcoholics; in O.A. Parsons, N. Butters and P.E. Nathan (eds), *Neuropsychology of Alcoholism: Implications for Diagnosis and Treatment*, Guildord Press, New York.

Goldstein, G., Ryan, C., Turner, S.M., Kanagy M., Barry, K. and Kelly, L. (1985) Three methods of memory training for severely amnesic patients, *Behaviour Modification*, **9**, 357–74.

Goldstein, G. and Ruthven, L. (1983) *Rehabilitation of the Brain Damaged Adult*, N. Yak, Plenum Press.

Goldstein; G. and Malec, E. (1989) Memory training for severely amnesic patients, *Neuropsychology*, **3**, 9–16.

Greene, J.G., Timbury, G.C., Smith, R. and Gardiner, M. (1983) Reality orientation with elderly patients in the community: an empirical evaluation, *Age and Ageing*, **12**, 38–43.

Hanley, I.G. (1981a) *An evaluation of reality orientation procedures with the mentally impaired elderly*, PhD thesis, University of Edinburgh.

Hanley, I.G. (1981b) The use of signposts and active training to modify ward disorientation in elderly patients, *Journal of Behaviour Therapy and Experimental Psychiatry*, **12**, 241–7.

Hanley, I.G. (1984) Theoretical and practical considerations in reality orientation therapy with the elderly; in I. Hanley and J. Hodge (eds), *Psychological Approaches to the Care of The Elderly*, Croom Helm, London.

Hanley, I.G. (1986) Reality orientation in the care of the elderly patient with dementia – three case studies; in I. Hanley and M. Gilhooly (ed), *Psychological Therapies for the Elderly*, Croom Helm, London.

Hanley, I.G., McGuire, R.J. and Boyd, W.D. (1981) Reality orientation and dementia: a controlled trial of two approaches, *British Journal of Psychiatry*, **138**, 10–14.

Harrington, D.L., Haaland, K.Y., Yeo, R.A. and Mardner, E. (1990) Procedural memory in Parkinson's disease: impaired motor but not visuospatial learning, *Journal of Clinical and Experimental Neuropsychology*, **12**, 323–39.

Harris, J.E. and Sunderland, A. (1981) A brief survey of the management of memory disorders in rehabilitation units in Britain, *International Rehabilitation Medicine*, **3**, 206–9.

Heindel, W., Butters, N. and Salmon, D. (1988) Impaired learning of a motor skill in patients with Huntington's disease, *Behavioural Neurosciences*, 102, 141–7.

Hendrich, D.W., Healey, A.F. and Brown, L.E. (1988) *Long term retention of procedural and episodic memory for digits*, paper presented at the 29th Annual Meeting of the Psychonomic Society, Chicago, Illinois.

Herrmann, D.J., Buschke, H. and Gall, M.B. (1987) Improving retrieval, *Applied Cognitive Psychology*, 1, 27–33.

Hersen, M. and Barlow, D.H. (1976) *Single Case Experimental Designs: Strategy for Studying Behaviour Change*, Pergamon, New York.

Hodge, J. (1984) Towards a behavioural analysis of dementia, in I. Hanley and J. Hodge (eds), *Psychological Approaches to the Care of the Elderly*, Croom Helm, London.

Kahn, R.L., Zarit, S.H., Hilbert, N.M. and Niederehe, G. (1975) Memory complaint and impairment of the aged: the effects of depression and altered brain function, *Archives of General Psychiatry*, **32**, 1569–73.

Karlsson, I., Brane, G., Melin, E., Nyth, A.L. and Rybo, E. (1988) Effects of environmental stimulation on biochemical and psychological variables in dementia. *Acta Psychiatrica Scandinavica*, **77**, 207–13.

Kovner, R., Mattis, S. and Goldmeier, E. (1983) A technique for promoting robust free recall in chronic organic amnesia, *Journal of Clinical Neuropsychology*, **5**, 65–71.

Kovner, R., Mattis, S. and Pass, R. (1985) Some amnesic patients can freely recall large amounts of information in new contexts, *Journal of Clinical and Experimental Neuropsychology*, 7, 395–411.

Kurlychek, R.T. (1983) Use of a digital alarm chronograph as a memory aid in early dementia, *Clinical Gerontologist*, **1**, 93–4.

Landauer and Bjork (1978) Optimum Rehearsal patterns and name learning, in M.M. Gruneberg, P.E. Morris and R.N. Sykes (eds) *Practical Aspects of Memory* London: Academic Press, 625–6.

Langer, E.J. and Rodin, J. (1976) The effects of choice and enhanced personal responsibility: a field experiment in an institutional setting, *Journal of Personality and Social Psychology*, **34**, 191–8.

Langer, E.J., Rodin, J., Beck, P., Weinman, C. and Spitzer, L. (1979) Environmental determinants of memory improvement in late adulthood, *Journal of Personality and Social Psychology*, **37**, 2003–13.

Lawson, M.J. and Rice, D.N. (1989) Effects of training in use of executive strategies on a verbal memory problem resulting from closed head injury, *Journal of Clinical and Experimental Neuropsychology*, **11**, 842–54.

Linton, M. (1988) The maintenance of knowledge: some long-term specific and generic changes. In M. Gruneberg, P. Morris and R. Sykes (eds), *Practical Aspects of Memory*: **1**, J. Wiley and Sons, Chichester.

Martone, M., Butters, N., Payne, M., Becker, J. and Sax, D. (1984) Dissociation between skill learning and verbal recogniton in amnesia and dementia, *Archives of Neurology*, **41**, 965–70.

McCartney, S.M. (1984) *Spatial orientation training in hospitalised patients with dementia*. Dissertation for the Diploma in Clinical Psychology, British Psychological Society, Leicester.

McCarty, D. (1980) Investigation of a visual imagery mnemonic device for acquiring face-name association, *Journal of Experimental Psychology: Human Learning and Memory*, **6**, 145–55.

Milner, B., Corkin, S. and Teuber, J.L. (1968) Further analysis of the hippocampal amnesic syndrome: a 14-year-follow-up study of HM, *Neuropsychologia*, **6**, 215–34.

Moffat, N.J. (1984a) Memory therapy with the elderly; in S. Simpson, P. Higson, R. Holland, J. McBrien, J. Williams and L. Henneman (eds), *Facing the Challenge*, British Association of Behavioural Psychotherapy, London.

Moffat, N.J. (1984b) Strategies of memory therapy; in B.A. Wilson and N.J. Moffat (eds), *Clinical Management of Memory Problems*, Croom Helm, London.

Moffat, N.J. (1989) Home based cognitive rehabilitation with the elderly; in L.W. Poon, D.C. Rubin and B.A. Wilson (eds), *Everyday Cognition in Adulthood and Late Life*, Cambridge University Press, Cambridge.

Raybould, E.C. and Solity, J. (1982) Teaching with precision, *Special Education: Forward Trends*, 9, 9–13.

Rea, C.P. and Modigliani, V. (1988) Educational implications of the spacing effect; in M.M. Gruneberg, P.E. Morris and R.N. Sykes (eds), *Practical Aspects of Memory: Current Research and Issues*, J. Wiley and Sons, Chichester.

Reeve, W. and Ivison, D. (1985) Use of experimental manipulation and modified informal reality orientation with institutionalised, confused elderly patients, *Age and Ageing*, **14**, 119–21.

Rodin, J. and Langer, E. (1977) Long-term effects of a control-relevant intervention among the institutionalised aged, *Journal of Personality and Social Psychology*, 35, 897–902.

Schacter, D.L., Rich, S.A. and Stampp, M.S. (1985) Remediation of memory disorders: experimental evaluation of the spaced retrieval technique, *Journal of Clinical and Experimental Neuropsychology*, 7, 79–96.

Shenton, R.K. (1975) The automatic memorandum clock. *Antiquarian Horology, June*, 337–9.

Squire, L. and Cohen, N. (1984) Human memory and amnesia; in J. McGough, G. Lynch and N. Weinburger (eds), *Neurobiology of Learning and Memory* (pp. 3–64), Guildford Press, New York.

Stigsdotter, A. and Backman, L. (1989) Multifactorial memory training with older adults: how to foster maintenance of improved performance, *Gerontology*, **35**, 260–7.

Vroman, G., Kellar, L. and Cohen, I. (1989) Cognitive rehabilitation in the elderly: a computer-based memory training program; in E. Perecman (ed), *Integrating Theory and Practice in Clinical Neuropsychology*, Lawrence Erlbaum Associates, Hillsdale, New Jersey.

Warrington, E. and Weiskrantz, L. (1974) The effect of prior learning on subsequent retention in amnesic patients, *Neuropsychologia*, 12, 419–28.

Wilson, B.A. (1981) Teaching a patient to remember people's names after removal of a left temporal lobe tumour, *Behavioural Psychotherapy*, 9, 338–44.

Wilson, B.A. (1984) Memory therapy in practice; in B.A. Wilson and N.J. Moffat (eds), *Clinical Management of Memory Problems*, Croom Helm, London.

Wilson, B.A. (1987) *Rehabilitation of Memory*, Guildford Press, London.

Wilson, B.A. and Moffat, N.J. (1984) Running a memory group; in B.A. Wilson and N.J. Moffat (eds), *Clinical Management of Memory Problems*, Croom Helm, London.

Wollen, K.A., Weber, A. and Lowry, D.H. (1972) Bizarreness versus interaction of mental images as determinant of learning, *Cognitive Psychology*, **3**, 518–23.

Zarit, S.H., Zarit, J.M. and Reever, K.E. (1982) Memory training for severe memory loss: effects on senile dementia patients and their families, *Gerontologist*, 22, 373–7.

Zencius, A., Wesolowski, M. and Burke, W. (1990) The use of a visual cue to reduce profanity in a brain injured adult, *Behavioural Residential Treatment*, 5, 143–7.

Zepelin, H., Wolffe, C.S. and Kleinplatz, F. (1981) Evaluation of a year-long reality orientation program, *Journal of Gerontology*, **36**, 70–7.

# Chapter 5

# Memory therapy in practice

## BARBARA WILSON

### THE NATURE OF MEMORY IMPAIRMENT

The reader of this chapter will be helped to plan and carry out memory therapy programmes for patients whose memory problems result from acquired brain damage.

Memory problems are commonly seen after many types of brain injury and if extreme are usually more handicapping in everyday life than severe physical problems. The most frequent causes of permanent organic memory impairment are

1. the degenerative disorders (particularly Alzheimer's disease)
2. severe traumatic brain injury (head injury)
3. Korsakoff's syndrome (associated with chronic alcohol abuse and poor nutrition)
4. brain surgery (such as that for intractible epilepsy or removal of a tumour or clipping of an aneurysm)
5. infections of the brain (for example, herpes simplex encephalitis or infection with Human Immunodeficiency Virus/HIV)
6. cerebral vascular disorders (particularly following a ruptured aneurysm on the anterior communicating artery)
7. anoxia or shortage of oxygen to the brain (perhaps following myocardial infarction or carbon monoxide poisoning).

These conditions are not of course mutually exclusive. It is possible, for example, to sustain a severe head injury and have anoxia, or to suffer brain damage from surgery that was required to clip an aneurysm. For the reader who wishes to learn more about these disorders Lishman (1987) and Kapur (1988) are recommended.

Although precise figures are not available, those working in the field are aware of the considerable numbers of memory-impaired people in society. We know that some 10% of people over the age of 65 years have dementia (Joynt and Shoulson, 1979) and some 36% of people surviving severe head injury will have significant memory problems (Schacter and Crovitz, 1977). Such figures mean that there will be about 2500 new cases of memory impairment from head injury each year in Britain and perhaps as many as 8000 or 9000 in the USA. When figures for dementia, Korsakoff's syndrome, encephalitis and other infections are added to these totals we can begin to appreciate the enormity of the problem facing communities.

As pointed out in Chapter 1, memory is not one unified skill or ability but consists rather of an overlapping range of 'sub-systems'. For this reason it is unlikely that any single solution will be found to help all people with memory difficulties; nor can we expect one strategy or technique to solve all the memory problems experienced by an individual patient. Given this scenario, how does a therapist decide where to begin treatment when a patient has been referred for help with memory problems?

We can assume that anyone working in the field will have gathered some understanding of the nature of human memory from the work of cognitive psychologists and neuro-psychologists who have studied normal human memory and the impaired memory functioning of patients with lesions in the central nervous system (Chapter 1 discusses these issues in some detail). The term 'amnesia' may be applied to a patient's memory difficulties. Amnesia means literally a lack or absence of memory, although in practice patients almost never forget everything: they usually remember how to walk, to talk, and the names of those they have known for a long time, as well as facts about their own autobiographies. Amnesia is better defined, then, as a failure in some part of the memory system. It remains nevertheless a confusing term because it is sometimes used to refer to problems experienced by people who have memory difficulties but no other cognitive problems and sometimes used much more loosely to refer to people with severe general intellectual deterioration which includes memory impairment.

To avoid misunderstandings of this kind, a diagnosis of the classic amnesic syndrome should be made only in people who have great difficulty learning and remembering information of nearly all kinds; who have a normal short term or immediate memory when this is measured by forward digit span and the recency effect in free recall; who have difficulty in remembering some information acquired before the onset of syndrome; and who also have normal or near normal functioning of other cognitive abilities. Although people with the classic amnesic syndrome are to be found, they are seen much less often than people who, in addition to experiencing memory problems, also have difficulties in reasoning, attention, word-finding and/or a slowing down of thinking and intellectual ability.

Whether a person has a 'pure' amnesia or more widespread cognitive impairments the typical picture of someone with organic memory problems is as follows

1. Immediate memory is reasonably normal.
2. Difficulties are experienced in remembering after a delay or distraction.
3. Learning of new material is difficult.
4. There is a tendency to remember things that happened a long time before an accident or illness better than things which happened a short time before.
5. Remembering how to do things that were previously well known and well practised may continue to be reasonably competent.
6. Cues, in the form of initial letters or rhymes or photographs of forgotten places may assist remembering.

### GENERAL PRINCIPLES FOR HELPING MEMORY-IMPAIRED PEOPLE

We learned in Chapter 1 that memory can be regarded as having three stages: input, storage and retrieval. There are researchers who argue that amnesia is basically a deficit in input, others who claim it is essentially a storage problem, and others who regard it as a retrieval deficit (Wilson, 1987, discusses these arguments in more detail). Baddeley (1982a and b) believes that none of these explanations are sufficient to explain all instances of the amnesic syndrome. We can nevertheless draw upon opposing research paradigms to provide guidelines for helping memory-impaired people, some of whom will have deficits at the input, storage or retrieval stages, others having deficits at more than than one of these stages.

The guidelines drawn up below are based on work carried out in cognitive psychology over the past 20 years or so. They will not of course *solve* memory problems experienced by brain-injured patients but may improve or ease situations in which brain-injured patients find themselves – particularly if those patients' impairments are relatively mild.

### GETTING THE INFORMATION IN

1. *Simplify* information we expect the brain injured person to remember. This applies particularly to the written word. For example, a head-injured person who needs to change the batteries in a piece of equipment that is used frequently may not be helped by reading 'Insert two R6 batteries checking the correct polarity.' (Actual example from a recently marketed device.) The instruction may be remembered better if it is written 'Put two R6 batteries plus to plus and minus to minus.'
2. *Reduce* the amount to be remembered (for example, ask the person to remember one thing rather than three things).
3. Make sure the brain-injured person has *understood* the information by repeating it back or re-telling in his/her own words.
4. Try to get the person to *link* the information to something s/he already knows, that is, to make associations. For example, the name of the therapist might be better remembered if it is associated with a relative or film star of the same name.
5. When assisting a brain-injured person to learn or remember something new use the rule of *'little and often'*. Generally, it is better to work at remembering something

a few minutes several times a day than for an hour once a day.

6. If possible, encourage the brain-injured person to *organize* the information that is to be remembered. We know, for example, that if people are asked to remember a shopping list they remember more when they group items into categories such as vegetables, dairy produce, stationery and cleaning materials than if they simply list items randomly.

## STORING THE INFORMATION

Most people forget new information rather rapidly over the first few days and then the rate of forgetting slows down. This is also true for people with memory problems, bearing in mind of course that in their case relatively little information gets stored in the first place. However, once we have helped get the information in we can help keep it there by testing or persuading the memory-impaired person to rehearse or practise it at intervals. The best way to help here is to test the person immediately after seeing or hearing the information, then test again after a short delay, then again after a slightly longer delay. This process is continued with the intervals being lengthened gradually. Such practice or rehearsal usually leads to better retention of information.

## RETRIEVING THE INFORMATION

It is sometimes the case that although one has learned something one just cannot 'reach' it when it is required. Obviously, this is more often experienced by a person with memory problems. If we can provide that person with a 'hook' in the form of a cue or prompt s/he may well be able to 'reach' the correct memory. Providing the first letter of a name may lead to the person remembering the whole name. Perhaps all of us have faced a situation where a face is recognized but not the name that goes with the face. This is particularly likely to happen if the person is seen in a different place from that in which an earlier meeting took place. Retrieval is easier for most of us if the surroundings in which we are trying to remember something are the same as those in which we first learned it. In the case of people with memory problems we may find they remember better if, when trying to remember something, they are in the same room with the same people as were there when that something was first learned or experienced.

It follows from this that when trying to teach a memory-impaired person new information we should aim to teach that person to remember that information in a number of different settings and social situations. Our aim should be to encourage learning in many different, everyday situations that are likely to be encountered in daily living. Learning must not be limited to a classroom or hospital setting.

The mood or state of mind we are in may influence our ability to remember. We know that people who learn things when they are sober remember them better when they are sober. Whilst this may not seem surprising, it is also true that things learned when a person is drunk may be better remembered when that person is drunk again. Similarly, things learned when one is happy or sad are better recalled when the original emotion is experienced. Consequently, when helping a memory-impaired person to remember we should aim to teach that person in a number of different moods.

Cues and prompts also help remembering, so sometimes we might supply the first letter or sound or part of a word to enable a memory-impaired person to find the information required. Sometimes it is possible to help people find their own prompts or cues by systematically going through letters of the alphabet ('does this person's name begin with A...B...C... etc.') Similarly, if a person has mis-laid something it often helps to go back to the last time that person remembers possessing the item, then ask the person to go through very carefully all the actions that followed. In this way the location of the lost article may be recalled.

Many patients referred for treatment will need help with problems that are either too specific or too severe to be assisted by the general guidelines above. Initially, brain-injured people with such problems will need detailed assessments to highlight their particular difficulties.


ASSESSMENT

Several memory assessment procedures are described in Chapter 2. It is important to remember that assessments should be carried out to build up a comprehensive picture of a person's functioning, and to see how that person's problems are manifested in everyday life.

A neuropsychological assessment, for example, may tell us whether a patient is intellectually impaired, whether the memory deficit is global or restricted to certain materials, whether recall and recognition are differentially affected, whether additional cognitive deficits are present, whether a score on any particular test is abnormal, and how the patient compares with peers. Whilst this is of course important information it is not the only kind of information required. A knowledge and understanding of ways in which memory problems are exhibited in daily living and how they affect the patient, the family and other carers is needed before one can offer assistance that will be genuinely helpful in daily routines, social intercourse or work situations. Is the patient ready and safe to return home or restart work? What are the main difficulties as perceived by the patient or family? What coping methods have been tried so far? In order to answer such questions some kind of behavioural assessment is necessary. Behavioural assessments can enable identification of particular problems experienced by the patient, they can measure the frequency and/or severity of these problems and they can evaluate the effectiveness of an intervention programme. For those readers unfamiliar with behavioural assessment Keefe, Kopel and Gordon (1978) is recommended as a simple introduction. Wilson (1987a) also discusses behavioural assessment in relation to memory rehabilitation.

Basically, a behavioural assessment should

1. Identify a problem as unambiguously as possible. ('Memory difficulty' would not, for example, be an

appropriate definition as it lacks specificity. 'Difficulty finding the way from the ward to physiotherapy' on the other hand would be acceptable).

2. Measure the deficit, that is, assess how often a problem occurs or how often a behaviour fails to occur, thus establishing a baseline against which the effects of treatment can be compared.
3. Set a target or goal, for example, teach the way from the ward to physiotherapy.
4. Select the most appropriate treatment.
5. Assess the ongoing treatment.
6. Evaluate therapy.

Most of these points will be discussed in the last sections of this chapter.

The Rivermead Behavioural Memory Test (Wilson, Cockburn and Baddeley, 1985) attempts to bridge conventional and behavioural procedures. This test requires patients to remember to carry out some simple, everyday tasks and to retain some information similar to that required for adequate everyday functioning. Originally designed for use with brain-injured patients between the ages of 16 and 65 years, the test now has norms for the elderly and for children. It has also proved useful for a wide range of neurological conditions including multiple sclerosis, Parkinson's disease, HIV infection, sub-arachnoid haemorrhage and early Alzheimer's disease.

IDENTIFYING PROBLEMS FOR TREATMENT

Once a detailed assessment has been completed it is possible to identify areas for treatment. When the first edition of this book appeared in 1984 the claim was made that therapists would receive little help from published accounts of attempts to improve the recall of brain-injured people. At that time most research concentrated on teaching lists of words or paired associates rather than identifying or treating practical problems experienced by memory-impaired people. The trouble with such research is that it very often fails to connect with the needs of the memory impaired, who in their daily lives are not bothered by the fact that they cannot remember paired associates or lists. Instead they want to remember what happened a few hours ago, where they left their belongings, whether they have taken their medication; they want to remember the names of their relatives and friends.

There were nevertheless some exceptions, in 1984, to the general practice of teaching things unrelated to the skills required for everyday living. For example, Sunderland, Harris and Baddeley (1983) gave a questionnaire to head-injured people and their relatives to discover the kinds of memory problems head injured people faced. As far as treatment was concerned Wilson (1982) described methods for treating a number of specifically identified problems. As there are now signs that more researchers are beginning to concentrate on practical issues it is hoped that therapists will gain considerably more help from the literature in the future than they have in the past.

Davies and Binks (1983) described the use of a prompt card to support the residual memory of a Korsakoff patient and Kurlychek (1983) reported the use of a digital alarm timer to remind a patient in the early stages of dementia to check his notebook. Since then more reports of work on real problems that make daily living for the memory impaired difficult have appeared. Amongst these are work by Glisky, Schacter and Tulving (1986), Wilson (1987a) and Moffat (1989).

Whilst such reports should enable therapists to develop understanding of the typical problems faced by memory-impaired people, a possibly more pressing concern for individual therapists is to determine the needs and develop specific programmes for each of their patients. A therapist can of course obtain information from interviewing a patient and the family. In certain cases patients specify their particular difficulties. One of my patients, for example, was very good at describing his main problems. He said he was unable to remember people's names or what day of the week it was. He had to look in his notebook when he was on the bus in order to recall his destination. He was a keen gardener but in order to retain a piece of information about gardening he had to read the same paragraph over and over again and even then he was likely to get details confused. With this man it was reasonably straightforward to decide areas on which to work. Other patients, however, refuse to admit they have any difficulties. They forget how forgetful they are. Others know they have problems but are unable to be specific when attempting to describe them. Many say something like, 'It's everything . . . I just can't remember anything.' When such a response occurs it is possible to go through a check-list or questionnaire. Several have been developed, for example, Bennett-Levy and Powell (1980) and Herrman and Neisser (1978). Probably one of the most useful questionnaires is that (described earlier) by Sunderland, Harris and Baddeley (1983). However, as the authors point out, filling in such a questionnaire is in itself a memory task so some memory-impaired people are not likely to be very accurate.

It is usually better to ask relatives or other staff closely involved with the patient to fill in the questionnaire or check-list. Sunderland *et al.* (1983) and Sunderland, Harris and Gleave (1984) have used both questionnaire and check-list with head-injured patients and their relatives in an attempt to see how often everyday memory problems occur and whether findings correlate with performance on standardized tests. The check-lists are filled in each evening for seven days. Those that have been produced by Sunderland *et al.* have been modified and adapted for therapists to use at Rivermead Rehabilitation Centre. Therapists fill in the list at the end of each session (there are five sessions a day) for each patient for a two-week period. This sounds very time-consuming and disruptive but in practice therapists find the task easy and much useful information has been gathered in this way. A sample of the 28-item check-list is illustrated in Table 5.1.

In addition to questioning the patient, relatives and staff the therapist should try to observe the patient in a variety of settings to see the kinds of problems which may occur. In the case of out-patients this might be difficult but in a hospital or rehabilitation unit one might be able to observe in occupational therapy, physiotherapy, in a memory group, or even at lunchtime. The observer should ask such questions as: 'Does the patient keep repeating

**Table 5.1** A sample page of the 28-item checklist

Date:——————  Day:——————

1. Did X forget where s/he put something? Did s/he lose things around the department?

2. Did s/he forget a change in her/his daily routine? For example, a change in the place where something is kept? Or a change in the time that something happens? Or follow an old routine by mistake?

3. Did s/he have to go back to check whether s/he had done something that s/he meant to do?

4. Did s/he forget when something happened? For example, whether it was yesterday or last week?

5. Did s/he forget to take things with her/him, or leave things behind and have to go back for them?

6. Did s/he forget that s/he was told something yesterday or a few days ago, and have to be reminded of it?

7. Did s/he ramble and speak about unimportant or irrelevant things?

8. Did s/he fail to recognize, by sight, close relatives or friends that s/he meets often?

9. Did s/he have difficulty in picking up a new skill. For example, in learning a new game or in working a new gadget afer s/he had practised once or twice?

10. Did s/he find that a word was 'on the tip of her/his tongue' and knew what it was but couldn't find it?

11. Did s/he forget to do things s/he said s/he would do?

Source: With permission from Alan Sunderland

the same story, question or joke? Does the patient forget instructions? Does the patient get lost on the way to the canteen?'

A further very important consideration for the therapist when selecting problems for treatment is the future vocation and destination of the patient once therapy has finished. The aims of treatment will be very different for someone who is hoping to take up a university place or return to a high-powered job than they will be for someone going to sheltered accommodation or into long-term care. Treatment

Session

| 9.00–10.30 | 10.45–12.00 | 1.30–2.30 | 2.30–3.00 | 3.15–4.30 |
|---|---|---|---|---|
| | | | | |
| | | | | |
| | | | | |
| | | | | |
| | | | | |
| | | | | |
| | | | | |
| | | | | |
| | | | | |
| | | | | |
| | | | | |

goals will be influenced by information from all the sources outlined above.

The next question the therapist may ask is: 'How many problems should be tackled at any one time?' There is no easy answer to this question. Circumstances will probably dictate what actually happens. The most intensive memory therapy I have undertaken was with Mr B, a 51-year-old man (whose treatment is described in detail elsewhere; see Wilson, 1982). Mr B had suffered a bilateral stroke which left him with a classic amnesic syndrome, that is, he had no physical, language or intellectual problems except with tasks involving memory. He received general memory stimulation five days a week for a period of six weeks. In addition, four specific memory problems were treated. These involved remembering his daily timetable, people's names, a shopping list and routes around the unit. Three of these were reduced by memory training strategies (different strategies being needed for each problem). The fourth, remembering short routes, remained resistant to all the approaches tried. Concurrently with this programme Mr B was making extensive use of his noteboook which contained details of his stroke, the consequences of this, what was happening at home and so forth. Notebooks are, of course, external aids and provide valuable help in reducing everyday problems. In effect, many of Mr B's problems were being dealt with simultaneously.

At the other extreme there are patients who are so impaired that almost everything is done for them. They are taken from one place to another and they may be unable to use external aids because of physical limitations, reading difficulties or sensory deficits. In these cases it is probably wiser to begin with one problem area, see what can be done, and extend the range of problems tackled when it is feasible.

With yet another group of patients it may be quite clear what is required of the memory therapist. For example, helping a patient to remember how to transfer from a wheelchair to an ordinary chair, or stopping a patient from repeating the same question over and over again, or encouraging a patient to refer to a notebook.

In this section I have attempted to show therapists ways of identifying problems for treatment. The next stage in memory therapy is to consider how to select the most appropriate treatment strategies for individual patients.

SUITING STRATEGY TO PATIENT

The strategies available to memory therapists have already been described in Chapter 4. It is not intended to describe the strategies again in this chapter but rather to suggest ways in which a therapist might arrive at a decision as to which strategies to use with different patients. With the exception

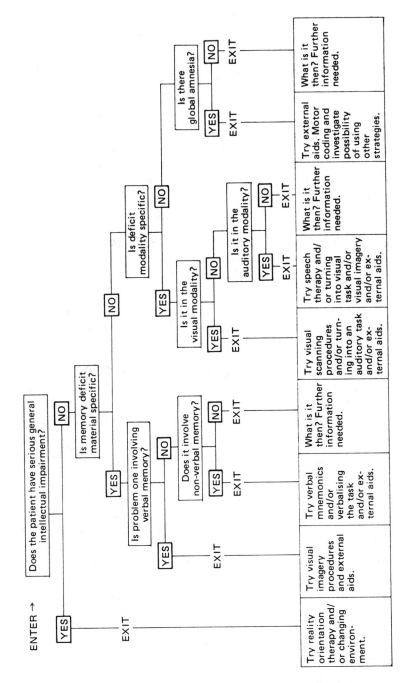

**Figure 5.1** Deciding on a treatment strategy for a memory impaired patient.

of Wilson and Moffat (1984a) there is little guidance in the published literature as to how to choose the appropriate strategy for a particular patient. Factors which influence whether anyone can use a certain technique depend, among other things, on the cause and site of brain damage, and the individual patient's style and preference.

The flow chart in Figure 5.1 offers one plan of action therapists might wish to follow in selecting a treatment strategy. Although I would not expect this plan to work every time for all patients and all problems it should be useful as a starting point. It may help therapists to clarify their own thoughts and trigger off further ideas.

For patients with general intellectual impairment therapists may find the best they can do is to make certain changes in the environment to enable patients to cope better with their handicap. Such changes include labelling doors, painting lines from one place to another or repositioning written material or objects so they will be more easily seen. Colour cues may also be used to provide extra information. Harris (1980a), describes, for example, how painting lavatory doors a different colour from all other doors reduced incontinence in one geriatric unit. Wilson (1981a) describes how coloured dots on visual symbol cards enabled one severely aphasic man to discriminate beteen confusing symbols.

Reality Orientation is another approach which can be considered (see Chapters 4 and 9 for more detailed analyses of Reality Orientation). As head-injured patients still in post-traumatic amnesia resemble, to some extent, the demented geriatric patients for whom Reality Orientation was initially developed, it might be advisable to attempt RO with the former group. Complete success cannot be guaranteed, however. At Rivermead I once tried RO with a young head-injured man still in post-traumatic amnesia. Before treatment I asked him where he thought he was and he replied 'It's Brackley School, isn't it?' He then went on to point out the English, Mathematics and Science departments. This was followed by three weeks of daily RO. At the end of this time I asked him where he thought he was now and he replied, 'Rivermead Rehabilitation Centre' but added, 'It's really Brackley School.'

As far as external aids are concerned some may be helpful for those with general intellectual deterioration. People who will benefit most from such aids, however, are those whose intellectual functioning is adequate but who have a specific memory deficit or a global amnesia. For these people external aids would appear to have a crucially important role to play in the rehabilitation of memory. Problems arise because it is not always easy to convince memory-impaired patients themselves of the importance of such aids. They may be unaware of the severity of their difficulties. They may see such aids as signs of weakness and argue that their memories will not improve if they rely on notebooks. Alternatively, they may simply forget to write down information or forget to check whether something is recorded. Counselling or instruction in the use of aids may be necessary in these cases. Sometimes it may be possible to change from one kind of aid to another. Take, for example, the case of a patient who refuses or is unable to remember to use a notebook. He or she may benefit from the provision of an electronic aid which has both an auditory signal (to act as a reminder to look at the aid) and a written message describing what has to be done.

Success may be achieved by replacing a written aid with a pictorial aid for an aphasic patient who is no longer able to read. One such aid was devised at Rivermead for an aphasic patient who could not learn how to transfer from her wheel-chair to her bed. (Figure 5.2 illustrates the aid.) The patient kept this pictorial representation with her and referred to it when transferring. The problem was not completely solved as she still needed observation during transfer. However, she transferred less dangerously than before and required less help from others.

A different pictorial system was employed with another globally aphasic patient who was referred four years after a stroke which left him unable to speak or understand single words at the level of a two-year-old. He was referred primarily because of stress at home. His wife was unable to communicate to him any changes in his daily programme. He spent several months learning a visual symbol system which soon helped his comprehension and to a lesser extent enabled him to express himself. Interestingly at this time the

TRANSFER

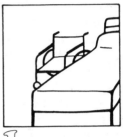 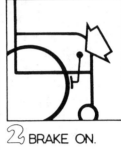 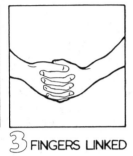

1 BRING THE CHAIR CLOSE TO THE BED

2 BRAKE ON.

3 FINGERS LINKED

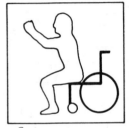 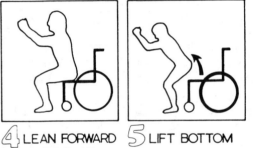 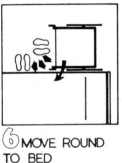

4 LEAN FORWARD EDGE OF CHAIR FEET LEVEL

5 LIFT BOTTOM

6 MOVE ROUND TO BED

7 LOWER BOTTOM DOWN SLOWLY

**Figure 5.2** A pictorial memory aid to help an aphasic patient remember how to transfer.

patient used his visual symbols to refer to events which had happened in the past or were to happen in the future. In other words, he was remembering by using the symbols. For example, one card depicted the following symbols:

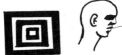

(Symbolizing the following)
Ben     sang (with)     Barbara     and     Philippa

The patient sometimes retrieved this card from the photograph album in which he kept the cards, pointed to it and then pointed to himself and Barbara or Philippa. It is probably rare for such a severely language impaired person to be able to refer to the past and future in this way.

No single external aid is likely to solve all the problems experienced by a memory impaired person. Different aids may be necessary for different tasks. For example, a wall calendar may tell a memory-impaired person the date of his next dental appointment but it is unlikely to contain information about how to get to the dentist's surgery. Given the importance of external aids, there are surprisingly few published accounts of such aids being used with memory-impaired people. Fowler, Hart and Sheehan (1972) used a small portable timer with a head-injured man so that he would remind himself to look at his timetable of daily events and move from one scheduled activity to another. The timer was gradually faded out. Klein and Fowler (1981) used a calculator with a built-in timer (the Casio PW.80) to remind paraplegics to lift from their wheelchairs regularly in order to prevent pressure sores. Wilson and Moffat's (1984b) dysarthric patient employed the same timer to remind himself to swallow saliva regularly. Kurlychek (1983) has already been mentioned. Sohlberg and Mateer (1989) describe the use of personal organizers with brain injured people.

In addition to the treatments described above there has also been some discussion by other interested parties concerning the potential application of external aids to the requirements of brain-damaged people. Jones and Adam (1979), for example, suggested using a microcomputer as a prosthetic memory. A small tape recorder would be included, containing instructions. Harris (1978, 1980b and Chapter 3 of this book) gives detailed accounts of the kinds of aids available (see also Chapter 6).

Unfortunately, all the electronic aids available have serious disadvantages for memory impaired people. In the first place they are expensive. It has proved impossible for many patients to learn how to programme them and even when the machines are pre-programmed by other people the user has to remember certain quite complicated steps (how to clear a screen and how to read messages already stored, for example). Such procedures are difficult for severely amnesic people to remember. Wilson and Moffat (1984b) provide further discussion on the advantages and disadvantages of various electronic aids. All we need add here is the hope that recent developments in microcomputers and calculators will in time benefit the brain-damaged population.

If a memory deficit is one primarily involving verbal memory and little else then visual imagery techniques should be seriously considered and their application investigated. As Moffat describes in the previous chapter, there are several visual imagery techniques and I will not refer to all of them here. The one I have employed most often, and most successfully, requires drawing a picture of a name which is to be learned. 'Stephanie' was drawn as a step and knee, and 'Dr Crossley' drawn as a cross leaf. Such examples worked well for patients with left hemisphere damage (Wilson, 1981a; Wilson and Moffat, 1984b) – including patients with mild aphasia. Some patients with right hemisphere or bilateral damage may be able to practise this technique although those with marked perceptual difficulties are unlikely to find it of much help (Wilson, 1987). I have even known a few patients who perform worse with visual imagery than with no strategy at all. The face-name association procedure is a variation on the theme already described. Non-brain-damaged people do best when all the steps of this technique are included (McCarty, 1980). Both Glasgow *et al.* (1977) and Wilson and Moffat (1984b) found that this was not true for certain brain-damaged people who were apparently unable to cope with all the face-name association stages. There are some who can benefit however so, along with other visual imagery procedures, it may be worth trying it out systematically with individual patients.

Some visual imagery techniques involve considerable verbal elements, one of them being the visual peg method described in Chapter 4. There are patients who can easily learn the verbal pegs but cannot remember the images placed in or on the pegs. Other patients cannot remember the pegs but once these are given they are able to recall the images with some degree of ease. Some patients with mild head injuries have learned to use the visual peg method in an experimental setting but practical, everyday applications may well be limited (although see Chapter 6).

Verbal strategies appear to work best for those with a reasonably intact language dominant hemisphere and whose memory problems are primarily of a non-verbal nature. Wilson (1982) described how a stroke patient was able to use a first-letter mnemonic to solve a spatial memory task. A PQRST strategy was employed with another patient in an attempt to prevent him asking the same question *ad nauseam*. (This strategy is described in Chapter 4: the letters standing for Preview, Question, Read, State and Test). This particular man, who had suffered a right hemisphere sub-arachnoid haemorrhage following rupture of an anterior communicating artery aneurysm, constantly asked the question: 'Why have I got a memory problem?' After several weeks of answering this question several times a day it was decided to teach him the answer by using a verbal memory-training technique. The patient wrote from dictation a summary of his illness, operation, resultant problems and prognosis. The PQRST technique was then operated with the patient selecting the key questions. The questions chosen were (a) What has happened to me? (b) When? (c) What was the result? (d) What are my main problems now? (e) How long will I be here at the rehabilitation centre? (f) What is the long-term prognosis? Each weekday for the next three weeks the patient was asked the selected questions at the beginning of each session. The correct answer was supplied if he failed to answer or answered incorrectly. This was followed by giving the patient the summary sheet and going through the whole PQRST strategy again. At the end of three weeks the man 'knew' the correct answers to most of the selected questions. The procedure was successful experimentally but not clinically, for in spite of nearly 100% correct responses when the therapist asked the questions the man still repeated his original question several times a day. It would appear that although he 'knew' the answer he could not or would not search his memory for the information. The situation is very like that described by Walsh (1978) when he wrote 'at other times frontal patients act as though they have lost the "strategies of recall" which enable them to utilise the information which they have already stored' (p. 319).

Wilson (1987) reports a series of studies using PQRST. The strategy was superior to rote rehearsal for almost all patients studied. It seems particularly valuable for head-injured patients who are able to remember at least one item from a prose recall task after an hour's delay without using a specific strategy. If they are 'off the floor' so to speak it appears that the PQRST has an opportunity to exert its influence. The major effect of PQRST is probably due to the fact that it requires a deep level of processing (Chapter 1).

For some non-verbal memory problems, such as difficulty in remembering the way from one place to another, it may be possible to teach patients to make the task a more verbal one by verbalizing the steps required. Thus, for example, instead of using spatial memory to find the way to the newsagent it might be possible to learn the following instructions: 'Go down the road towards the big white building. Look for the telephone box and turn down the road next to it. Look for the house with the yellow door, and the newsagent's shop is two doors further on.'

As well as problems with specific material (that is, verbal or non-verbal), some people encounter difficulty in certain modalities or when the material is presented in a certain way. Sometimes, then, the memory problems may be restricted to the visual modality. In the former, patients are unable to remember much of what they see and in the latter they remember little of what they hear. If the memory deficit is modality rather than material specific other treatment techniques may be needed. Those patients who demonstrate problems in the visual but not the auditory modality may have a unilateral spatial neglect or visual scanning problem, and may need treatment to improve their scanning. Diller and Weinberg (1977) describe some methods used successfully to reduce hemi-inattention. Alternatively, it may be possible to change the task from a visual to an auditory one either by describing the material to the patient or teaching the patient to verbalize the material.

When problems occur in the auditory but not the visual modality it is possible that speech therapy is required as this pattern may occur with language disorder. If a language disorder is not present it may be possible to teach the patient to change the task from an auditory to a visual one by visualizing or drawing information as much as possible.

The final treatment approach to be discussed here is motor coding or using movement as a memory aid. It has been established that the motor memory of amnesic patients is less impaired than many other aspects of memory (e.g. Brooks and Baddeley, 1976). An interesting question for memory rehabilitation is whether we can capitalize on this intact ability in order to ameliorate deficits caused through impairment of other memory systems. There is no conclusive answer at present but partial success has been achieved with one severely amnesic young man treated at Rivermead. MC had been presented with many treatment strategies, on an individual basis and within a group. He remained disoriented in time and place and was unable to identify any of the people who had treated him for the past two years. Several attempts were made to teach him the names of people with whom he regularly came into contact. Visual imagery failed but he learned to associate ten signs with names. He chose most of the signs himself, pretending for example to eat soup for 'Sue', and sniffing a rose for 'Ros'. If the sign was demonstrated to him he reliably recalled the name with which it was associated. If one of the ten people concerned said 'What's my name?' and made the appropriate sign he gave the correct answer. He could not, however, reliably pair the sign with the correct person if several people or several photographs were placed in front of him and the sign not given. His difficulty is confounded by a face-recognition problem. Nevertheless, he learned to pair signs with names and, perhaps, for a person with a severe amnesia without perceptual problems, movement as a memory aid may turn out to be effective.

USING MEMORY STRATEGIES IN REHABILITATION

It is unrealistic to expect most memory-impaired people to be able to use memory strategies spontaneously. Ideally we would like to teach a strategy to a person and then expect that person to employ the strategy every time s/he needs to remember something, but this is beyond the capabilities of most memory-impaired people who are likely to forget the contents and/or sequence of the strategy. Many memory-impaired people have additional cognitive difficulties which affect their ability to plan, organize or initiate adequate problem-solving procedures. This does not mean the strategies are useless but rather that they are not panaceas. The following guidelines are offered to those intending to teach memory strategies (particularly internal kinds).

1. Internal strategies can be used to teach some new information (Wilson, 1987) although they will not be taken on board and used spontaneously.
2. Dual coding is usually better than single coding (Paivio, 1969; Wilson, 1987). If the memory-impaired patient wants to learn and retain something there is a greater chance of success if two methods of remembering are used rather than one. For example, if the number of a bank service card needs to be remembered, the method whereby each digit is turned into a word containing the same number of letters could be tried. Thus the number 4355 could become 'Don't(4) eat(3) stale(5) bread(5)'. The method of expanding rehearsal could also be employed to learn the phrase/number. Triple or even quadruple coding methods can be taught so that, in our example, a visual image could be formed of somebody pushing away stale bread, or the number 4355 might be thought of in terms of, say, the patient's house number (43) and the date in which his first car was bought, say, '55.
3. Teaching should proceed one step at a time. A typical study looking at visual imagery in the 1970s would

attempt to teach 15 words in three trials to a group of control subjects and a group of brain-injured people; the control subjects would benefit from imagery, the brain injured subjects would not. The researchers would therefore conclude that brain-injured people were not helped by visual imagery. Obviously, such a procedure was unhelpful for the brain-injured subjects who were not given a sufficient number of steps or time in which to assimilate the knowledge being offered. After all, no serious teacher of, say, a mentally handicapped child would attempt to teach 15 items in three trials. In this respect cognitively impaired people need as much thought going into ways they are taught as do mentally handicapped children.

4. It is better to draw images than to rely upon mental imagery. Evidence suggests that it is more effective for either the patient or therapist to draw images for visual imagery procedures than to expect the patient to carry the image mentally. This remains true when the patient understands what is required and is quite capable of forming a mental image. The very mildly impaired may be equally good at benefiting from drawn and mental images but the moderately and severely impaired show superior performance with drawn images (Wilson, 1987).

5. Material to be learned should be realistic and relevant to the needs of the patient. Here again early studies which attempted to improve the recall of brain-injured patients by using experimental material ran into difficulties that could have been avoided had the information been recognized as helpful by the patients. Patients have sufficient difficulties learning to cope with everyday problems and generalizing from specific learning material to real life situations: they do not need their mental systems cluttered up by extraneous material. We should teach real names and real routes in real situations.

6. Therapists should also recognize that individual patients have individual styles and preferences when it comes to learning. Not everyone will like visual imagery or first letter mnemonics even though such strategies have proved effective with some. The position is even more complex when we recognize that one procedure may be

preferred for one particular problem but not another. Visual imagery, for example, may be a good way of learning names but less good for learning a shopping list. Flexibility and ingenuity are likely to remain the therapist's best attributes.

## HOW TO TEACH THE STRATEGIES

Having decided what problems to tackle and what strategies to use in an attempt to ameliorate them, the next step is to consider how best to teach the strategies. A behavioural approach to memory rehabilitation is recommended because

1. it is adaptable to a wide range of patients, problems and settings;
2. the goals are small and specific;
3. assessment and treatment are inseparable;
4. treatment can be continuously and easily monitored and
5. there is evidence that suggests that this approach can be effective (e.g. Wilson, 1987; Moffat, 1989).

A behavioural programme for the treatment of a memory-impaired person should be organized in the following stages:

1. Specify the behaviour to be changed. 'Inability to learn people's names' or 'Difficulty in remembering short routes' would be appropriate ways of describing problems. Vague and general descriptions such as 'Impaired concentration' are unhelpful.
2. State the goals or aims of treatment. Again, these should be as specific as possible. Appropriately expressed aims would read like the following: 'To teach Mrs A the way from the ward to physiotherapy', 'To teach Mr B to check his notebook every half-hour' or 'To determine whether method A or method B is better for improving recall'.
3. Measure the deficit in order to obtain a satisfactory baseline. This can be achieved in several ways. Examples are: 'by recording how often Mr C repeats the same question in a week' or 'how many times in a given period of time Mrs D forgets to put her wheelchair brakes on before transferring.

All the recording methods employed in behavioural assessment and treatment are of potential use. It may also be necessary to carry out a more detailed analysis of factors affecting memory failures. For example, does stress make the problem worse? Is relaxation training indicated? Does it help to pace information, that is, present it at a slower rate? Does extra rehearsal improve matters? What happens if the material to be learned is written down? What happens if another person presents the information?

4. Decide on the most suitable treatment strategy for the particular individual. (Suggestions in the previous section may help here.)
5. Plan the treatment. The following questions will provide guidance for the therapist through this stage (although it may not be necessary to go through *all* of these questions in each particular case):
   (a) What particular strategy should be used?
   (b) Who is to do the training?
   (c) When is the training to be carried out and where?
   (d) How is it to be conducted and how often?
   (e) What happens if the patient succeeds in remembering the task?
   (f) Will such success be sufficient reward in itself?
   (g) Will some further reinforcement be required?
   (h) How will you measure success?
   (i) What happens if the patient fails at a task?
   (j) In the event of such failure is the patient to be reminded, ignored, or shown the correct way?
   (k) Who will be responsible for keeping records? Will it be the therapist, the patient, the family or an independent observer?
6. Begin the treatment.
7. Monitor and evaluate progress according to the plan outlined in Stage 5.
8. Change the procedure if necessary.

These guidelines will be familiar to people involved in designing behaviour modification programmes; fewer people will be aware of their application to the field of memory rehabilitation. Table 5.3 is an example of a successful programme for a man who was unable to find his bed on the ward.

**Table 5.3:** Programme to teach Mr J to find his bed

| | | |
|---|---|---|
| 1. | Specify behaviour | Mr J. cannot find his way round ward. |
| 2. | State aims | Teach Mr J. to find his own bed. |
| 3. | Measure deficit | Failed on six consecutive occasions. (Went to wrong bed twice. Asked staff four times.) |
| 4. | Decide on treatment strategy | External aids/environmental modifications. |
| 5. | Plan treatment | 1. Red notices placed at head and foot of Mr J.'s bed. 2. Mr J. to be given a card stating his bed third from the door with red notices at head and foot. 3. Signs and arrows pointing to Mr J.'s bed from door, from toilet and or wall above bed. |
| 6. | Monitor and evaluate | No more errors – Mr J. always found own bed. |
| 7. | Change procedure if necessary | 1. Remove signs and arrows. See if Mr J. can manage with card and red notices. 2. Teach Mr J. the way to the toilet using a similar procedure. |

Throughout this chapter there has been some emphasis on the teaching of names. As well as highlighting techniques which can be applied to other problem areas, names are important in themselves. Inability to remember names is one of the most frequent complaints found among memory-impaired patients so they *want* to learn them. In addition, it is usually possible for therapists to find a way of teaching at least a few names. Finally, because patients achieve some degree of success in this area they may be encouraged to apply successful strategies to other problems.

Other principles from behavioural psychology which have a part in memory rehabilitation include shaping, chaining, prompting and modelling. Shaping, or gradually working towards the final goal, is a long-established procedure which has some limited value in memory training. Chaining is a useful and adaptable technique for teaching new skills and would appear to have much to offer memory rehabilitation. It involves breaking down any piece of behaviour into a series of steps or links in a chain. Only one step is taught at a time. Once the first step has been learned the second is added then the third and fourth and so on. (See Yule and Carr, 1987 for a more detailed description of this procedure.) Chaining has been used at Rivermead to teach patients to remember how to transfer from wheelchairs to ordinary chairs. Usually the physiotherapist works out the necessary steps. An example of this would be the following:

1. Position wheelchair correctly.
2. Check brakes are on.
3. Remove feet from foot rests.
4. Move bottom forwards.
5. Position feet correctly.
6. Position arms correctly.
7. Lean forward.
8. Lift bottom.
9. Swing bottom towards seat of the chair.
10. Move feet and straighten up.

If forward chaining is the method chosen then the patient is expected to complete the first step unaccompanied. Once this is achieved the therapist reminds or guides the patient through each successive step. In *backward* chaining the reminding or guiding is carried out up to the last step, which the patient is expected to complete unaided. When the patient is able to do this the preceding step is attempted and so on until the first step is tackled. Although backward chaining is probably used more often in mental handicap there is no evidence to suggest which of the two is more effective as a teaching technique. Indeed, choice may depend ultimately on the nature of the particular task being learned.

Schacter and Glisky (1986) and Glisky, Schacter and Tulving (1986) have used a chaining procedure to teach amnesic patients to use computers. Although the authors called the procedure 'the method of vanishing cues' it is identical to the well-established backward chaining procedure from behavioural psychology.

Prompting is another useful behavioural procedure for the memory therapist. Physical, verbal and gestural prompts can be used, either on their own or in combination. The prompts are gradually faded out as the subject becomes more able to manage alone. Physical prompting may prove useful in teaching a memory-impaired person new skills. For instance, working a machine will require guidance through the task at the start with the therapist providing less and less physical prompting as the trainee becomes more adept.

Jaffe and Katz (1975) used verbal prompting and fading to teach a Korsakoff patient two names. this man had not learned anyone's name in five years of hospitalization. He was told: 'This person's name is Paul Doty, try to remember the initials P. and D.' The next time P.D. was introduced as Paul D. and the patient asked to supply the full name. The verbal cues were gradually reduced and two names were learned in this way over a period of two weeks. A somewhat similar procedure was introduced at Rivermead to teach a young head-injured woman the correct month, to help her overcome her disorientation in time. Songs were used as verbal prompts. In June the song chosen was 'June is busting out all over.' The next time the young woman was asked the month and gave an incorrect answer she was asked, 'What song did we have?' and she was able to supply the correct answer. Over the next two days the cue was reduced to 'What song?' then 'Song?', after which she reliably said 'June.'

Modelling, or learning from imitating others, has been used with phobic patients and obsessive compulsives. It may also have an important part to play in memory training. A modelling technique was employed to teach a severely aphasic man some limited communication skills (Wilson 1981a). It may also be of value in persuading some memory-impaired people to use notebooks and other external aids. If they see other people with similar problems making use of such aids they may be more willing to employ them. From research on modelling we know that people are more likely to imitate peers than someone less like themselves.

Also they are more likely to imitate people with high than with low prestige. Sex, age, social class, ethnic status and the competence of the model are other influencing factors (Carr, 1987). Active participation leads to better results than passive observation of others, and live models are better than filmed ones. All these findings can be incorporated into memory-training programmes and may be particularly pertinent for the organizers of memory groups.

This is not a fully exhaustive list of teaching methods. Other techniques such as self-instruction may prove equally useful in some cases. Moffat (Chapter 4) describes these in detail. The role of computers, drugs, external aids and group training are discussed elsewhere in this book. Finally, the motivated and interested therapist may be able to find new methods from other fields and other disciplines which can be adapted for the benefit of memory-impaired people.

## GENERALIZATION

Whilst we can provide memory-impaired people with memory aids or strategies to assist in overcoming their identifiable memory problems at the time they receive therapy, there is no guarantee that these aids or strategies will be employed by patients in their daily lives outside the context of immediate rehabilitation. Indeed the likelihood is that a great number of techniques will be forgotten by patients once they leave the rehabilitation unit. Sometimes the memory-impaired person will use a strategy or aid for one problem but not make use of that same strategy or aid for another problem equally suited to its application. Similarly, a strategy may be exercised in one situation but not in another equally relevant situation. These omissions do not mean the strategy or aid itself is of no value. After all, we do not call a hearing aid useless if a partially hearing person refuses to wear it. What we need to do, however, is find ways to ensure the hearing aid is worn. Similarly we need to ensure that transfer or generalization of rehabilitative techniques takes place *outside* the context of our teaching programmes.

We can begin by recognizing that generalization will not occur spontaneously with brain-injured people in general or memory-impaired people in particular. However, it is possible to teach generalization in some circumstances. This is accepted by teachers of people with a mental handicap (Zarkowska, 1987) who recognize that skills learned in the classroom must be accompanied by generalization programmes if those skills are going to be exercised in the home. A generalization programme can follow a similar procedure as that presented in Table 5.3. The aim might be to teach a patient to use a notebook in (1) speech therapy, (2) on the ward, and (3) at home during weekends. The treatment plan might involve the use of a timer to remind the patient to look at the notebook, or to have a reminder from a speech therapist, nurse or parent. The reminders will be faded out across the different situations listed above.

In many cases it is sensible to build in generalization from the beginning of a programme. Mr A, for example (Wilson, 1981), was taught to remember his therapists' names by using imagery in the form of a drawing of each name. As described earlier, the name Stephanie was represented by a step and knee. Apart from initial sessions when the images were introduced, the team of therapists began generalization training straight away. The first step was to vary the setting in which learning took place so various rooms were used throughout the centre. Next, the therapists themselves called in during various sessions so that Mr A, could address them by name, and finally Mr A. was accompanied round the rehabilitation centre to meet therapists in their own rooms.

An essential part of the rehabilitation of a memory-impaired person, in order to ensure generalization, is the teaching of people who will have most contact with the patient in everyday situations. These will include staff, friends and family. It was explained, for example, to Mr A's wife that if he needed to learn the name of a new neighbour or colleague she should ask her husband to draw a picture of the name, rehearse this several times a day, and arrange meetings with the neighbour or colleague in a variety of contexts. It was also pointed out that names should be learned one at a time in order to avoid confusion.

A final point which needs stressing is that we should not stop teaching new information to severely memory impaired people simply in the belief that generalization will not occur.

Such an outlook would indeed be defeatist and would lead memory therapy into a cul de sac from which there would be no turning. Any successful learning, however limited it is to a specific context, is a step forward for a severely impaired person. Schacter and Glisky (1986), for example, taught some of their patients the commands necessary to operate a computer by the method of vanishing cues. The method itself did not stay in the minds of the patients but some nevertheless learned to use a computer. Thus the strategy was a means to an end, however limited that end might be in space and time. Similarly, visual imagery, first letter mnemonics, expanding rehearsal, PQRST and other strategies can be the means to specific objectives: that is, we can teach some new information more effectively using memory strategies than we can without using them. Achievements are thus possible. It is up to us to extend and increase the contexts in which achievements can occur.

## REFERENCES

Baddeley, A.D. (1982a). Amnesia: A minimal model and an interpretation. In: L. Cermak (ed.), *Human Memory and Amnesia*. Lawrence Erlbaum Associates, Hillsdale, New Jersey.

Baddeley, A.D. (1982b). Implications of neuropsychological evidence for theories of normal memory. *Philosophical Transactions of the Royal Society London B*, **298**, 59–72.

Bennett-Levy, J. and Powell, G.E. (1980). The subjective memory questionnaire (SMQ): an investigation into the self-reporting of 'real-life' memory skills. *British Journal of Social and Clinical Psychology*, **19**, 177–83.

Brooks, D.N. and Baddeley, A. (1976). What can amnesics learn? *Neuropsychologia*, **14**, 111–22.

Carr, J. (1987). Imitation. In W. Yule and J. Carr (eds), *Behaviour Modification for People with Mental Handicaps* (pp. 95–101) Croom Helm, London.

Davies, A.D.M. and Binks, M.G. (1983). Supporting the residual memory of a Korsakoff patient. *Behavioural Psychotherapy*, **11**, 62–74.

Diller, L. and Weinberg, J. (1977). Hemi-inattention in rehabilitation: the evolution of a rational remediation program. In E.A. Weinstein and R.P. Friedland (Eds.), *Advances in Neurology*, **18**. Raven Press, New York.

Fowler, R., Hart, J. and Sheehan, M. (1972). A prosthetic memory: An application of the prosthetic environment concept. *Rehabilitation Counselling Bulletin*, **15**, 80–5.

Glasgow, R.E., Zeiss, R.A., Barrera, M. and Lewinsohn, P.M. (1977). Case studies on remediating memory deficits in brain damaged individuals. *Journal of Clinical Psychology*, **33**, 1049–54.

Glisky, E.L., Schacter, D.L. and Tulving, E. (1986). Computer learning by memory impaired patients: acquisition and retention of complex knowledge. *Neuropsychologia*, **24**, 313–28.

Harris, J.E. (1978) External memory aids, in *Practical Aspects of Memory*, M.M. Gruneberg, P. Morris and R. Sykes (eds), Academic Press, London.

Harris, J.E. (1980a). Memory aids people use: Two interview studies. *Memory and Cognition*, **8**, 31–8.

Harris, J.E. (1980b). We have ways of helping you remember. *Concord. The Journal of the British Association for Service to the Elderly, No. 17*, 21–7.

Herrmann, D. and Neisser, U. (1978). An inventory of everyday memory experiences. In M.M. Gruneberg, P. Morris and R. Sykes (Eds.), *Practical Aspects of Memory*. Academic Press, London.

Jaffe, P.G. and Katz, A.N. (1975). Attenuating anterograde amnesia. *Journal of Abnormal Psychology*, **84**, 559–62.

Jones, G. and Adam, J. (1979). Towards a prosthetic memory. *Bulletin of the British Psychological Society*, **32**, 165–7.

Joynt, R.J. and Shoulson, I. (1979). Dementia. In K.M. Heilman and E. Valenstein (eds), *Clinical Neuropsychology*. Oxford University Press. New York/Oxford.

Kapur, N. (1988). *Memory Disorders in Clinical Practice*. Butterworths. London.

Keefe, F.J., Kopel, S.A. and Gordon, S.B. (1978) *A Practical Guide to Behavioural Assessment*, Springer Publishing Co., New York.

Klein, R.M. and Fowler, R.S. (1981). Pressure relief training device: the microcalculator. *Archives of Physical and Medical Rehabilitation*, **62**, 500–1.

Kurlycheck, R.T. (1983). Use of a digital alarm chronograph as a memory aid in early dementia. *Clinical Gerontologist*, **1**, 93–4.

Lishman, W.A. (1987). *Organic Psychiatry: The Psychological Consequences of Cerebral Disorder*. 2nd edition. Blackwell's Scientific Publications. Oxford.

McCarty, D. (1980). Investigation of a visual imagery mnemonic device for acquiring face-name associations. *Journal of Experimental Psychology, Human Learning and Memory*, **6**, 145–55.

Moffat, N. (1989). Home based rehabilitation programmes for the elderly. In L. Poon, D. Rubin and B. Wilson (eds), *Everyday Cognition in Adult and Later Life* (pp. 659–80). Guilford Press, New York.

Paivio, A. (1969). Mental imagery in learning and memory. *Psychological Review*, **76**, 241–63.

Schacter, D. and Crovitz, H. (1977). Memory function after closed head injury: A review of the quantitative research. *Cortex*, **13**, 105–76.

Schacter, D.L. and Glisky, E.L. (1986). Memory remediation: restoration, alleviation and the acquisition of domain-specific knowledge.

In B.P. Uzzell and Y. Cross (eds), *Clinical Neuropsychology of Intervention* (pp. 257–82). Martinus Nijhoff, Boston.

Sohlberg, M.M. and Mateer, C. (1989) Training use of compensatory memory books: a three stage behavioural approach, *Journal of Clinical and Experimental Psychology* **11**, 871–91.

Sunderland, A., Harris, J.E. and Baddeley, A.D. (1983). Do laboratory tests predict everyday memory? A neuropsychological study. *Journal of Verbal Learning and Verbal Behavior*, **22**, 341–57.

Sunderland, A., Harris, J.E. and Gleave, J. (1984). Memory failures in everyday life after severe head injury. *Journal of Clinical Neuropsychology*, **6**, 127–42.

Walsh, K. (1978). *Neuropsychology: A Clinical Approach*. Churchill Livingstone, Edinburgh.

Wilson, B.A. (1981a). A survey of behavioural treatments carried out at a Rehabilitation Centre for stroke and head injuries. In G. Powell (ed.), *Brain Function Therapy*. Gower Press, Aldershot.

Wilson, B.A. (1981b). Teaching a patient to remember people's names after removal of a left temporal lobe tumour. *Behavioural Psychotherapy*, **9**, 338–44.

Wilson, B.A. (1982). Success and failure in memory training following a cerebral vascular accident. *Cortex*, **18**, 581–94.

Wilson, B.A. (1987). *Rehabilitation of Memory*. Guilford Press. New York.

Wilson, B.A., Cockburn, J. and Baddeley, A.D. (1985). *The Rivermead Behavioural Memory Test Manual*. Published by Thames Valley Test Co., 7–9 The Green, Flempton, Bury St Edmunds, Suffolk.

Wilson, B.A. and Moffat, N. (1984a). *Clinical Management of Memory Problems*. Croom Helm, London.

Wilson, B.A. and Moffat, N. (1984b). Rehabilitation of memory for everyday life. In J. Harris and P. Morris (eds), *Everyday Memory: Actions and Absentmindedness*. Academic Press, London.

Yule, W. and Carr, J. (1987) (eds), *Behaviour Modification for People with Mental Handicaps* (Second Edition). Croom Helm, London.

Zarkowska, E. (1987). Discrimination and generalisation. In W. Yule and J. Carr (eds), *Behaviour Modification for People with Mental Handicaps* (pp. 79–94). Croom Helm, London.

*Chapter 6*

# Computer assistance in the management of memory and cognitive impairment

## CLIVE SKILBECK and IAN ROBERTSON

### INTRODUCTION

**Advantages of microcomputers.**

Microcomputers have been widely available for less than 10 years. During this period their cost has fallen significantly, although their storage capacity and flexibility has increased. The relatively high cost of IBM machines, and the limited availability of relevant compatible software, originally constrained their adoption for cognitive assessment and rehabilitation work. However, the introduction of much cheaper IBM-compatible micros has led to the increased popularity of this type of system; for example, an Amstrad 1640 system, including 20 megabyte hard disk, is available through the NHS for approximately £850. The spread of inexpensive IBM-compatible micros has, in turn, stimulated the rapid development of appropriate software, and the Journal of Cognitive Rehabilitation now lists programmes for IBM as well as for other machines. Both Commodore and BBC micros are commonly used in clinical settings in the UK, but the most popular machine on both sides of the Atlantic remains the Apple.

Clinical Psychologists were originally slow to exploit the potential of micros, although they are now increasingly found in Clinical Psychology departments where they are mainly employed for their data storage statistical analysis, and word-processing functions. The aim of this chapter is to outline the general case for using micros in the management of memory dysfunction, to offer a brief literature review, and to provide some illustrative clinical examples. The general case for employing micros in the clinical setting is very strong, and rests on a number of points:

## Cost time-saving considerations

Clinical neuropsychologists are a scarce resource, although they have a key research/evaluation role in the remediation of cognitive deficits and the provision of a rehabilitation service. Given that micros are cheap, delegation to the computer of only a small proportion of a psychologist's patient contact time, involving either memory assessment or treatment, makes its purchase cost-effective. This can free time for the psychologist to accept more referrals, which is particularly relevant in the neuropsychology specialty where there is high degree of face-to-face contact.

Space (1981) pointed to the dramatic reduction in 'turn-around' time between assessment and report delivery when a micro is employed to offer a battery of tests, automated scoring, computerized interpretation, and 'hard copy' report writing. Use of a micro may also mean that a psychology technician, rather than an additional clinical neuropsychologist, can be included in an expanding department. Sanders (1985) argued that greater efficiency can result from involving the micro in the decision-making regarding the number of items of a test to administer. He investigated the possibility of reducing the number of items of the Minnesota Multiphasic Personality Inventory (Dahlstrom, Welsh and Dahlstrom, 1975) which necessarily had to be administered to generate the 'full' inventory results. The results obtained, via multiple regression analysis, indicated that the number of test items could be reduced from 566 in the original version to 187, without significant loss of descriptive power: correlation between computer-predicted raw scores and actual raw scores had a mean of 0.95, with a range of 0.88–0.98. Similarly, profile prediction was very good (mean r=0.97). Replication of this type of work with other psychometric tests, and with new tests developed with the aid of micros, could produce significant time, and therefore cost, savings.

Besides being inexpensive, micros are highly reliable and virtually maintenance free: repair/service costs should be negligible.

## Provision of standard/controlled conditions

Micros offer the potential advantage of providing higher reliability for some psychological tests, by reducing/removing the variability which is inevitably introduced into their administration by human assessors. An important issue in neuropsychology is the assessment of progress or outcome following treatment. There is a need to interpret 'recovery' data – has any noted improvement resulted from spontaneous recovery, the specific therapy used, or because of uncontrolled factors? In this area, too, micros can assist in evaluation by allowing the standardized, controlled, presentation of test items and recording of patient responses.

## Flexibility

Micros can change the execution of a program whilst it is running. This can be extremely useful in the area of memory therapy. For example, if a patient who is receiving orientation training via computer (see below) correctly answers a test item on consecutive trials, the micro can be pre-programmed to omit that item on subsequent trials. Similarly, if an item proves too difficult, the micro can re-present it in an easier form. Such adjustments might be very difficult when face-to-face, given the necessity of preparing materials beforehand. Micros might be programmed with more sophisticated decision rules regarding cessation of testing than are currently possible with human test administration. For example, there are 'discontinue testing' WAIS-R (Wechsler, 1987) rules provided for clinical psychologists, but the internal computing speed and multiple-comparison capacity of micros could allow the latter to 'decide' to stop testing (according to rules provided by psychologists) in other test situations where the psychologist would have found the decision difficult (because of speed and complexity factors).

## Production of timed responses

Time measures have often been utilized to assist in the identification of brain damage. In recent years the apparatus employed has increasingly been computer-based. For example, De Mita, Johnson and Hansen (1981) described a visual search task, based on a DEC 11-series minicomputer, to discriminate between brain-damaged and non-brain-damaged people (86% 'hit' rate), and between people with brain damage and those with a psychiatric diagnosis (71% 'hit' rate).

It can be argued that the accurate timing of a patient's response latencies is very useful in assessing the success of cognitive rehabilitation. Timed measures may be more sensitive than accuracy alone to the process of cognitive recovery. There is some evidence to suggest that an improving visual reaction time performance may offer an early sign of improvement in the attentional deficit noted frequently in patients who have suffered a severe head injury (Skilbeck, 1989).

## Patient acceptability

Although the available research is limited, there is no evidence to suggest that a patient will respond less favourably via a computer than in a personal interaction. Indeed, patients may prefer its non-judgemental approach. Angle, Hay, Hay, and Ellinwood (1977) noted that a majority of their clients preferred computer to human interview in relation to a behavioural assessment. Lucas (1977), too, in a study of patients' attitudes to interview via computer demonstrated that 82% were well-disposed towards it, almost half preferring it to that conducted by a doctor. Carr, Ghosh, and Ancill (1983), investigating the obtaining of psychiatric histories from patients using micro interview, found a 90–93% accuracy compared with the information gathered by the psychiatric team. In addition, 88% of the patients found micro interrogation to be as easy as clinical interview, and for most of the patients the computer interview uncovered relevant items of information that were not known to the psychiatric team. Gedye and Miller (1970) reported that some elderly patients who had refused traditional testing accepted a computer version; a lack of interference from interpersonal and social factors may make computer-administration a very attractive technique for patients relearning a skill.

## Ease of data analysis

Once a patient has answered the computer's items, an immediate print-out of the responses and descriptive statistics (e.g., mean, standard deviation, appropriate norms) can be obtained. The patient's results can also be 'written' on to computer disk for permanent storage and future analysis. Space (1981) and Morris (1985) both pointed out that this function can be linked to automated clinical 'profiling', report generation, and prediction/prognosis. The process of accruing clinical norms is greatly assisted by an accumulating database.

## Disadvantages of microcomputers

Space (1981) has reviewed the possible arguments against using computerized assessment, including

1. micro systems depersonalize the patient;
2. micro-based evaluation is not sensitive to idiographic aspects of a patient's performance, only to characteristics related to nomothetic information;
3. psychodynamic analysis of performance is not possible;
4. neither the clinician, nor the patient, feels they can control the situation;
5. micro assessment systems are inflexible, unable to be sensitive to patient response style by shifting focus;
6. with difficult-to-assess patients, micros have little to offer, similarly with patients who may experience distress during interview/testing;
7. issues of cultural bias in testing, confidentiality, and protection of privacy are greater with micro involvement;
8. employment of micros in the testing situation introduces bias.

Clearly point 1. assumes a total absence of human interaction which should not be the case. As for the process of dialogue between micro and patient, the available evidence argues against a 'depersonalizing' effect. An example is provided by the work of Lucas (1977), referred to above. Also, Angle *et al.* (1977) observed a majority preference amongst patients for micro interview, and Slack and Slack (1977) noted improved reliability of the information gained via micro interview over that gleaned by a physician.

Micro evaluation can be designed along idiographic (ie, focused upon the individual and his/her personal uniqueness), rather than normative, lines. For example, Cliffe (1985) described the successful computerization of the Personal Questionnaire Rapid Scaling Technique (Mulhall, 1980), pointing out at the same time that patients found it more pleasant and clinicians gained time and ease of use from its employment. The program was written for an ITT 2020 micro, though it will run on Apples as well. Whilst there is continuing discussion regarding the validity of the 'idiographic' approach, there is no problem in principle regarding provision of this type of assessment using a micro; appropriate research and development is, however, required.

Employment of a micro does not, at the time of its use, facilitate psychodynamic evaluation. However, efficient use of cognitive assessment can free some additional clinician time to gain 'richer' psychological information. Clinicians can retain control of the micro use by either programming the computer themselves or directing the design of the software by computer scientists. The close co-operation of the clinician in the production of software may also improve flexibility by designing in desirable extra 'clinical' features.

The criticism based on difficult to assess/distressed patients is an important one. On the one hand the small amount of information which does exist tends to indicate that patients who refuse traditional testing sometimes will accept micro-based assessment (e.g., Gedye and Miller, 1970). Also, Moffat (1989) employed BBC micros with very withdrawn demented patients and noted these patients do respond at least as well using the machines as in face-to-face interactions. However, it is true that some behaviourally disturbed patients will be difficult to assess with a micro (although this applies also to traditional approaches). The area where most care should be taken is in employing micros to administer procedures (cognitive or questionnaire) that might provoke undue distress in patients. This latter point requires good clinical judgement and appropriate monitoring of the patient's experience of the micro-based evaluation. Other points relating to privacy, confidentiality, and bias are no greater than in traditional settings (and in some ways are easier to control).

Another possible risk is that the micro will 'take over' and be too influential in the psychologist's thinking with regard to the most appropriate tests and retraining procedures to employ; i.e., if the procedure is not machine-compatible, then do not bother to develop it. Linked to this is the problem of programming addiction, in which the psychologist continues to produce new programs which 'might be useful at some time', or is unable to leave a completed program alone, adding further options/refinements in a time-consuming manner. Possibly the most important issue is that the psychologist may come to employ tests and procedures merely because their use has been made possible by the introduction of micros, without due consideration of the implications from psychological theory.

### APPLICATIONS IN THE MANAGEMENT OF COGNITIVE/ MEMORY IMPAIRMENT.

Micros can assist in the management of cognitive/memory disorders by helping

1. to assess the deficit;
2. to measure the effectiveness of any intervention (e.g., drug therapy);
3. in the treatment procedures themselves.

### Assessment

In the future, micros will hold a key position in clinical and educational assessment. For clinicians one of the early important contributions was that of Acker (1980), whose battery is commercially available for the Commodore PET and C64, and for the Apple, from NFER-Nelson. The battery includes visual memory, verbal memory, symbol digit, visuospatial, and right-left orientation tasks, using its own button-press

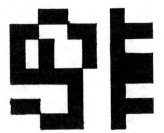

**Figure 6.1** Visual memory stimulus.

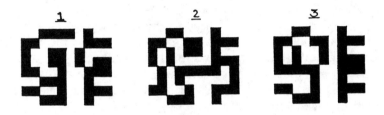

**Figure 6.2** Visual memory multiple choice response.

response keyboard to overlay the micro keyboard. Practice items are included for each test.

The visual memory task includes items which are impossible to code verbally, unlike some other clinical memory tests such as the Benton Visual Retention Test (Benton, 1974), and employs a multiple-choice response format. Figures 6.1 and 6.2 provide an illustration.

In the verbal memory task individual item exposure is followed by a multiple-choice recognition test. The symbol digit task is very similar to the digit symbol subtest of the WAIS-R, the major differences being that in the former symbols have to be translated into number responses (rather than vice versa), and the patient's responses take the form of pressing the appropriate button number to match each presented symbol rather than manually drawing the response. Accuracy and speed print-outs are provided for the first 20, middle 20, and final 20 trials separately, to provide a check on any fatigue or 'warm-up' factors that may be operating. For the visuospatial analysis items the patient is presented with three designs, two of which are identical, and has to find the 'odd man out'. The test includes two levels of difficulty, uses very similar material to that employed in the visual memory test, and employs the same multiple-choice recognition format. On each of Acker's tasks the print-out of results contains data on both accuracy and response latency.

Other micro test batteries are still rare, although Moerland, Alderkamp and De Alpherts (1986) developed one which runs on the Apple II-e. The battery still requires some active participation by a psychology technician or clinical psychologist, and a number of the tests are adaptations of traditional neuropsychological measures (WAIS-R digit span, Halstead-Reitan finger tapping and Seashore rhythm tests). However, most of the tests involve memory and attentional processes: both simple and two-choice reaction time tasks are included, as is an iconic memory task. The vigilance task chosen displays eight characters on the visual display unit (VDU) screen for a pre-determined number of trials and the patient has to identify the random position of the letter 'A'. Moerland *et al.* used a modification of the search task developed by De Mita *et al.* (1981), mentioned above, which draws heavily upon attention. The patient's task is to identify one grid pattern (of 24 in a numbered 'checkerboard') that matches the one displayed centrally on the VDU. Perhaps the most immediately relevant tests for clinical practice are the two short-term memory/learning tasks. The first parallels the Corsi block-tapping test (described in Lezak, 1983), the patient's response for the block sequence being recorded by means of a light pen. The second is a 15-word learning task which utilizes five trials and which can be presented in either auditory or visual modality. The task involves free recall on each trial, plus delayed recall after 15 minutes. Moerland *et al.* (1986) admitted that the obvious lack of normative information has initially restricted clinical interpretation, but they are accumulating relevant data. Interestingly, these authors commented on the lack of any specific resistance to micro testing, and recommended that institutions should co-operate (on cost grounds) for future program development.

Another attempt at establishing a collection of tests on micro was that of Beaumont and French (1987). Rather than constructing a battery, these authors developed modifications of traditional clinical psychology tests to run on Apple

II+ micros with touch-sensitive screens. The project was very ambitious, taking in five clinical establishments and 367 patients (only 73 of whom were 'definitely/possibly' neurologically impaired). The design included comparison of standard and micro test versions, and of keyboard versus 'touch' response methods. Included in the tests studied were Raven's Progressive Matrices (Raven, 1983), WAIS digits, Wisconsin Card Sorting Test (described in Lezak, 1983) and Money Road Map Test (Money, 1976). The results obtained from Raven's PM indicated that the traditional administration produced significantly ($p<0.005$) higher scores than the micro presentation, probably due to poor resolution of the computer graphics according to Beaumont and French. The reliability between traditional and keyboard versions (0.81) and between traditional and 'touch' versions (0.87) compared well with that available in the literature for the test-retest reliability of the traditional version.

Similar findings of the micro-based version yielding significantly lower scores than the traditional version were also noted in relation to WAIS digits, although no differences between keyboard and 'touch' response styles were observed. The correlations between traditional and micro-administrations were low for digits forward (0.56), though higher for digits backwards (0.71), and total (0.73) (relatively low test-retest reliability for the original version has been noted in earlier studies). Beaumont and French concluded that the automated digits task was not a psychometric parallel of the WAIS original. Their results for the Money Road Map Test yielded more acceptable reliability data, including a co-efficient of 0.83 for 'touch' and traditional versions. As the original manual offers no reliability information, it is impossible to set this result in context. However, the micro version led to a higher number of errors ($p<0.05$) and was slower to complete. Whilst concluding that automated parallel versions of traditional tests are feasible, Beaumont and French also recommended that future micro test development should introduce more 'intelligence' into the assessment systems.

Instead of investigating micro versions of traditional, psychometric, tests, some authors have produced tasks specifically designed for micro running. Schlichting and Wray (1986) described a system (Hewlett-Packard 85) which presented five different tests, including short-term memory, choice reaction time (RT), mental arithmetic, and a digit symbol substitution task. Listings and a floppy disk are available from the authors, and the system has the research and clinical advantages that the H-P 85 is highly portable for use in patients' homes. Another collection of tests examining memory performances is that produced by Algarabel (1983), which runs on Apple II. The collection involves free-recall, paired-associate, serial learning, and recognition experiments.

Rather than investigating/developing a battery, or collection of tests, most researchers have studied one task. A number of these will be briefly described, to reflect their variety. The value of the visual research task in identifying brain damage, developed by De Mita *et al.* (1981) has already been pointed out above. A program called 'FactRetrievel' has been produced by Shimamura, Landwehr and Nelson (1981) to run on Apples. The program presents up to 240 general knowledge questions, drawing upon the Nelson and Narens (1980) norms. The task involves three aspects – recall, feeling of knowing for non-recalled facts, and recognition of non-recalled facts. The recall aspect includes questions such as 'What is the capital of Chile?' Items from this section which a patient is unable to recall correctly are used in pairs in the second part, the patients deciding which one they feel they are more likely to recognise as correct. The final section consists of an eight-alternative forced-choice recognition task for each non-recalled item from the first section. The correlation between scores in section 2 and 3 offer a validity measure for patients in respect of 'feeling of knowing'. The program listing, or diskette, are available from the authors at the University of Washington, USA.

Ryan (1986) described a micro game ('memory for goblins') specifically designed to assess and train working memory. The program runs on Apple Micros and is described in the section below on cognitive rehabilitation. Finally, Calistri and Kallman (1986) reported on an automated diagnostic rhyme test developed for the Commodore 64. The program, available from the authors in New York requires a subject to recall/identify which of two visually-presented words matches the word he/she has already heard.

### Measuring the effects of a therapeutic intervention

As mentioned earlier, the timing of response latencies is a particular feature of micros. The timing can be made very accurate, and it is easy to convert the machine to act as a millisecond timer by means of a short program. An example case study, using a Commodore PET, involved a patient (KW) who suffered a right frontal lobe haemorrhage, with subsequent neurosurgical intervention to clip the causal aneurysm. Repeated testing suggested that KW's cognitive functions had stabilized in the three months following his operation, leaving him with marked memory and learning deficits as evidenced by the Rey Auditory Learning Test (see Lezak, 1983) and Weschler Memory Scale Factor Scores (Skilbeck and Woods, 1980). In conjunction with a neurosurgeon, it was decided to use desmopressin (DDAVP) on an experimental basis with KW, there being some research to suggest its potential usefulness following brain injury.

After baseline testing, KW, was assessed approximately every two weeks for three months, alternately 'on' and 'off' the drug. Testing included visual RT measures of memory scanning, using a paradigm well known in experimental psychology (Sternberg, 1969). The design involved providing K.W. with a number of digits (the 'positive' set), and then presenting single digits to him visually through the VDU. On each trial, KW was required to press one response key if the presented digit belonged to the positive set, and another response key if it did not (ie a 'negative' set digit). For each assessment, K.W. was tested under four conditions of positive set size (1, 2, 3 or 4 digits). Figure 6.3 depicts the mean RT results for the four positive set size conditions, of each testing session. It can be seen that the plots for set sizes 1, 2 and 3 all show beneficial effects from the 'standard' dose of the drug, in terms of faster memory scanning. In contrast, plot 4 failed to show consistent changes according to drug condition. Also, when the drug dose was doubled, plots 1 and 2 deteriorated (point 6).

Although the results obtained were not totally consistent, they do suggest that medication may have some role in the amelioration of deficits in at least one area of memory functioning. The deleterious effects noted from doubling the drug

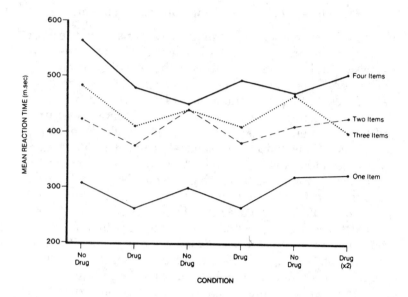

**Figure 6.3** Patient K.W.: mean RT and drug administration.

dose highlight the careful experimental work that is required in the field of drug effects and cognitive performance. Although in this case the micro was not directly involved in the process of remediation, it did prove a useful tool in assessing the beneficial effects of the 'memory drug'.

Another case example where the micro has proved useful in assessing cognitive change is that of T.A., who was a head-injured patient almost four years post-trauma when first seen. Unwittingly, T.A. was still taking a 100 mg daily dose of Phenytoin, on which he had been placed prophylactically immediately after his injury. Rather than just stop the anticonvulsant medication immediately, a baseline measure of his memory scanning performance with the existing level of medication was obtained. The drug dose was then halved and two weeks later he was reassessed. Finally, he was seen a further two weeks later, after he had been off medication for two weeks. Figure 6.4 shows T.A.'s median RT performances under increasing memory load (ie, with positive set sizes 1–4, according to Sternberg's paradigm;

Sternberg, 1969). On his original dose, T.A.'s performances were both slow and somewhat erratic. When the medication dose was halved, his performances generally were faster and the shape of the RT graph became nearer to that expected from a normal individual. Two weeks after he ceased taking Phenytoin altogether his performances were both fast and displayed a normal shape.

### Cognitive rehabilitation

In a major review article, Kurlycheck and Levin (1987) offered a critique of the use of micros in cognitive reha-bilitation. These authors started by considering the poss-ible processes involved in spontaneous recovery, and then contrasted two models of cognitive (re-)training. The first, basic skills training, is a neuropsychological/cognitive model which advocates that attention should centre on the underly-ing cognitive processes which are hypothesized as necessary to achieve the longer term acquisition of the skill under investigation. The other, direct skilled training model is more behavioural, being focused upon the specific functional skill that is to be (re-)trained. Kurlycheck and Levin suggested that the latter model may be less appropriate for severely impaired patients, in whom even simple functional skills probably require breaking down into small component steps comprising the skill (ie, analysis according to underlying cog-nitive processes). Kurlycheck and Levin indicated a number of elements which should be taken into consideration in any general paradigm of cognitive (re-)training, including:

1. Presenting tasks in sequence from simple to complex
2. Selecting tasks of a difficulty level that ensures a high rate of success
3. Requiring demonstration of mastery as a prerequisite to advancing
4. Emphasizing not just accuracy of response but rate or speed of response
5. Providing frequent positive or corrective feedback
6. Gradually decreasing or fading prompts by the trainer
7. Requiring increasing initiative and sustained endurance by the subject

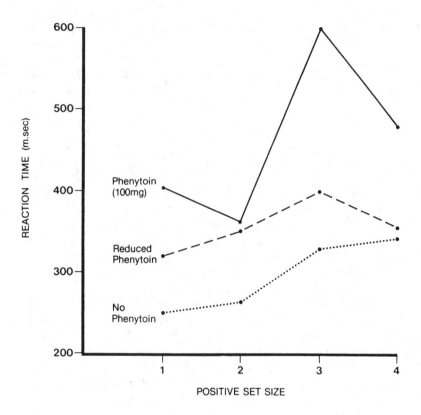

**Figure 6.4** Patient T.A.: median RT and medication level.

These elements are highly compatible with micro-based training.

Micros can be employed in 'orientation' memory re-training, an application which may be appropriate for patients who have sustained severe damage following head injury or stroke. The application originated in the field of psychogeriatrics, where a common problem is the 'confused' patient, deriving from Reality Orientation Training (ROT). As its name suggests, ROT focuses upon improving a patient's level of orientation (Holden and Woods, 1982), generally by giving frequent reminders to patients of items of information that should be familiar to them. Many neurological patients manifest similar difficulties in orientation, and from the therapy viewpoint a major problem in trying to reorientate patients is that techniques such as ROT are time-consuming. Rarely does a psychologist, or one of the other therapists working with the patient, have the time available to improve a patient's level of orientation; however, this long and monotonous aspect of memory retraining can largely be delegated to a micro. It is relatively easy to write a program that involves the micro asking patients orientation questions of personal relevance. Each question can be presented on the VDU screen, along with a number of possible answers. These answers are numbered, and the patient's task is to press the button number corresponding to the answer which he/she believes to be true. For this purpose, the patient is provided with a response board containing the numbered buttons which fits over the micro's usual keyboard to prevent the patient inadvertently 'crashing' the program. With this arrangement, it has been our experience that the large majority of neurological patients can comprehend the task instructions and follow the system.

The 'reorientate' computer program is written so that each time it runs it first requires the insertion of the orientation questions and possible responses. This allows flexibility in the retraining system (so that different orientation questions can be used, as appropriate), and also allows the psychologist to vary the number of items to be included on any particular run. Patient boredom is unlikely to occur. The method does not require that the same question has to be re-entered every time it is used at a particular session: the program is written so that it loops round and round to present the item a number of times, the number of 'loops' being determined by the psychologist on each occasion that the program is run. Maintenance of the patient's attention can be aided in a number of ways: for example, attention to the question presented can be maintained by adding an underlining to the question shortly after it has been displayed. Attention can be further enhanced by flashing the underlining off and on, or varying the colour in which the question is presented. Retraining of orientation via micro can be made far more interesting for the patient than the corresponding face-to-face interaction with the psychologist or therapist! Overloading the patient with a sudden appearance of a screen full of alternative responses to a question can be avoided by temporally sequencing their appearance on the screen. The patient should then be able to 'take in' the information more easily. Another potential problem that can easily be avoided is that of 'positional effects' operating on response selection. By the simple insertion of two lines of programming, the order in which the alternative responses are presented to the patient can be randomized. As is the case with the interpersonal retraining of orientation, it is important to provide the patient with feedback to reinforce selection of the right response, or correction of the wrong response. A number of feedback statements, therefore, need to be included in the program. Those confirming the correct response might include 'you are right', 'that is correct', or 'yes!', followed by a restatement of the correct response, and those when a wrong answer has been chosen might be 'don't forget', and 'try to remember', followed by the correct answer. Obviously a time limit has to be set, so that if the patient fails to respond within, say, ten seconds, the micro automatically provides the correct answer. It is relatively straightforward to write the program so that questions which the patient finds very easy (that is, always answers them correctly and speedily) can be omitted on later 'loops' of the program. Similarly, items that a patient finds too difficult can be omitted or re-presented in an easier form.

In addition to reducing the tedium for the psychologist, or therapist, who has frequently to repeat these orientation items, using a micro has a further advantage of providing accurate measurement of response latency. The ease with which a patient retrieves an item from memory can thus be gauged, as can the beneficial effects of preventing a particular item a number of times. Finally, the micro can provide a 'hard copy', or permanent record of the patient's reorientation sessions without detailed notes being necessary.

This type of program has been used with a number of patients in our unit who have memory and orientation difficulties. The data produced from our studies of these patients indicates shorter response latencies and greater accuracy, both between sessions and between trials within

**Table 6.1** Patient RM: Mean response latency (sec.) across sessions

|  | Session (Week) | | | | |
| --- | --- | --- | --- | --- | --- |
|  | 1 | 2 | 3 | 4 | 5 |
| Repeated questions | 4.1 | 2.8 | 2.8 | 2.0 | 0.8 |
| New questions | 2.4 | 3.2 | 2.8 | 2.5 | 2.5 |

**Table 6.2** Patient RM: Mean response latency (sec.) within sessions

|  |  | Trial | | | |
| --- | --- | --- | --- | --- | --- |
|  |  | 1 | 2 | 3 | 4 |
| Session (week) | 1 | 6.3 | 2.8 | 2.1 | 1.7 |
|  | 2 | 5.4 | 2.2 | 1.9 | 2.5 |
|  | 3 | 4.3 | 2.1 | 2.2 | 1.9 |
|  | 4 | 4.1 | 2.7 | 1.3 | 1.2 |
|  | 5 | 2.3 | 2.3 | 1.3 | 1.4 |

the one session. An example case is that of RM. RM was a longstanding severely head-injured patient when first seen for therapy. He had major memory and orientation difficulties. Using the program 'reorientate' he was given twenty-one orientation questions (on four repetition loops each session); over a number of weeks. The questions were divided into seven items which were repeated at each session (for example, 'Which famous politician died in 1989?'), seven questions which related to current news items, and seven questions which related to recent personal information. RM ran through the orientation program weekly, results obtained demonstrating that his mean response latency for repeated items decreased over the weeks (Table 6.1), and within a session (Table 6.2).

RM's accuracy of performance using micro-administered questions was compared with his results in a more traditional face-to-face orientation retraining. Very similar results were obtained in the two conditions with repeated items (Table 6.3), and for items which changed week to week (Table 6.4). Our results with RM show that learning does take place across trials in any particular session, and across sessions. Although the amount of data available is still limited, our findings do not suggest that major differences should be expected between micro-administered and face-to-face orientation retraining. The computerized condition offers the benefits of a non-judgemental approach and economy in terms of time spent in face-to-face treatment.

Johnson and Garvie (1985) discussed the BBC Micro as an aid in cognitive rehabilitation because of its use in occupational therapy departments in the UK. In addition to highlighting some general points in favour of using micros in cognitive rehabilitation, including patient acceptability and flexibility of programs, these authors addressed some of the factors which need to be borne in mind when designing programs. In their opinion, commercial programs are only appropriate for the more mildly brain-damaged patients, given that they usually require good recall of instructions, short response latencies and/or complex responses. Johnson and Garvie pointed out that for patient use instructions have to be brief, clear, and constantly available as reminders. Often patients are slow to learn how to use response devices and appropriate feedback on performance should be provided immediately. The difficulty level of a a program needs to be tailored to suit the capacity of an individual patient, either through built-in options or via alternative versions of the software. As indicated in the 'advantages' section of this chapter, flexibility can be designed into a program so that the

**Table 6.3** Patient RM: Orientation errors for repeated questions

|         |   | Computer trials | | | | Non-computer trials | | | |
|---------|---|---|---|---|---|---|---|---|---|
|         |   | 1 | 2 | 3 | 4 | 1 | 2 | 3 | 4 |
| Session | 1 | 7 | 3 | 1 | 0 | 7 | 2 | 1 | 0 |
|         | 2 | 4 | 2 | 1 | 0 | 4 | 1 | 1 | 0 |
|         | 3 | 6 | 0 | 0 | 0 | 0 | 0 | 0 | 0 |
|         | 4 | 0 | 0 | 0 | 0 | 0 | 0 | 0 | 0 |
|         | 5 | 0 | 0 | 0 | 0 | 0 | 0 | 0 | 0 |

**Table 6.4** Patient RM: Orientation errors for new questions

|         |   | Computer trials | | | | Non-computer trials | | | |
|---------|---|---|---|---|---|---|---|---|---|
|         |   | 1 | 2 | 3 | 4 | 1 | 2 | 3 | 4 |
| Session | 1 | 6 | 3 | 0 | 0 | 10 | 4 | 2 | 0 |
|         | 2 | 4 | 3 | 0 | 0 | 7 | 4 | 0 | 0 |
|         | 3 | 7 | 2 | 2 | 0 | 9 | 4 | 1 | 0 |
|         | 4 | 6 | 1 | 0 | 0 | 6 | 1 | 0 | 0 |
|         | 5 | 9 | 7 | 2 | 3 | 7 | 3 | 1 | 0 |

micro will alter the stimulus material it presents in the light of a patient's responses. Johnson and Garvie (1985) made a plea for the proper evaluation of cognitive rehabilitation software, given that it can be time consuming and expensive to produce and therefore a waste of resources if it is not beneficial to patients. Johnson and Garvie advocated the evaluation of any demonstrated therapeutic effects from the laboratory or clinic in terms of its generalization to real-life settings, and offered the opinion that using the micro to adapt or compensate for a lost ability is likely to prove more profitable than attempting restoration of the lost function. These authors advocated that linkage should occur between assessment of a patient's cognitive strengths and deficits and the subsequent attempt at micro-based rehabilitation.

Wood and Fussey (1987) undertook a controlled study of micro-assisted cognitive treatment using a Commodore C64. The experiment utilized three samples (N= 10 for each) – a severely head-injured group who received micro cognitive rehabilitation, a mixed (predominantly head-injured) group who received non-micro based cognitive rehabilitation, and a normal control group matched for age with patients. The cognitive therapy was targeted upon attentional/information processing deficits, with outcome being gauged via pre- and post-measures (including RT, vigilance, and verbal short-term memory and learning tasks). The post-test consisted of two assessments, one carried out immediately following the 20-day treatment program and one carried out a further 20 days later to allow estimation of the persistence of any demonstrated improvement. The only training task employed was visual and was directed at information processing ability with symbol material. It tapped visual scanning, perceptual discrimination, judgement and anticipation, vigilance, and RT performance, providing feedback on successful and error performance. The speed of running of the program was automatically adjusted by the micro as the patient showed training 'gain'. Each of the 20 training sessions comprised 60 minutes. The results for the micro cognitive rehabilitation group reflected a significant trend of improvement ($p<0.01$) on the training task over the first seven days of the program, though not subsequently. Interpretation of these findings are difficult, however, given

the changing task demands 'day by day'. Improved performances at post-test follow-up were also noted in relation
to RT speed and vigilance, and evidence of generalization
of improved attentional performance was also obtained
from rehabilitation therapists on other tasks ($p < 0.05$). The
improvements noted were not reflected in changes in cognitive test scores, although it may be argued that given
the difference in modality (training was exclusively visual,
cognitive tests were all verbal), and cognitive functioning
(cognitive tests were short-term memory or learning in
nature), such wide generalization was probably too much
to expect. However, Wood and Fussey's paper represents a
welcome attempt at vigorous investigation of micro cognitive
rehabilitation by means of a controlled experiment.

Finlayson, Alfano and Sullivan (1987) argued that a prerequisite for the successful application of cognitive rehabilitation procedures is a detailed description of the range
and severity of deficits. Their case study of cognitive
rehabilitation, therefore, was accompanied by a comprehensive neuropsychological examination and treatment plan. A
micro rehabilitation program was designed along the conceptual lines proposed in the REHABIT model (Reitan Evaluation
of Hemispheric Ability and Brain Improvement Training;
Reitan 1979). The patient undergoing therapy was a severely
head-injured woman who was 10 months post-trauma,
and micro based rehabilitation extended across a 22-week
period. The micro exercises involved visual RT, planning and
sequencing events in space and across time, visual digit span,
and two tasks simulating visuomotor control and judgement. The tasks under training were reported as showing
improvement over the rehabilitation period, and a number
of WAIS and Halstead-Reitan test scores (Lezak, 1983) also
showed gains. Finalyson *et al.* viewed the improvements in
neuropsychological test performance as 'strongly suggesting
the generalization of microcomputer-based improvements to
independent test performance'. This assertion seems open
to question, given that cognitive recovery, without targeted
rehabilitation effects, can be observed more than a year
post-trauma and the baseline assessment of their patient was
carried out at only 10 months post injury (van Zomeren and
Deelman, 1978). It is also difficult to view large improvements

in WAIS similarities and Halstead-Reitan category task and grip strength scores as stemming from the described micro training.

Kerner and Acker (1985) carried out an experimental study involving 24 head-injured patients (mild and severe) all of whom were at least 3 months post-trauma. Their computer memory retraining group (CMRG, N=12) received treatment using an Apple II+ Micro and employing Gianutsos and Klitzner (1981) software. This group's time on the micro in memory rehabilitation was matched by a computer control group (CCG, N=6) who engaged in the generation of graphics and pictures using the micro. Finally, the 'no exposure' control group (NECG, N=6) received neither treatment nor any micro exposure. Kerner and Acker used pre- and post-treatment Randt memory test scores (Randt, Brown and Osborne, 1980) as the measure of outcome. For the CMRG and CCG groups, 12 micro sessions of 45 minutes each were provided, over approximately one month. Kerner and Acker were interested in investigating efectiveness of micro memory training, the generalization of such training, and the maintenance of any gains achieved. The results they obtained demonstrated that the CMRG showed significant gains over the 12 sessions on the training tasks (P<0.001, P<0.0001) and between pre-test and 30-day post-test on the Randt memory test measures (P<0.0025, or better), thereby suggesting generalization of the effect. The gains of the CMRG over this period were significantly higher than for the CCG and NECG groups in terms of Randt acquisition and recall scale scores (P<0.01, P<0.10, respectively) and Randt memory index scores (both P<0.01). CCG and NECG results did not differ significantly from each other. However, Kerner and Acker noted losses between the 30-day post-test and 45-day post-test for the CMRG on three out of the four Randt measures. The authors indicated that 'lowered motivation' over the 15-day extra follow-up period might account for this finding, and advocated a longer period of retraining with a larger number of sessions to reinforce the acquired memory skills. It is also worth noting that change scores are compared for the different groups without baseline scores being reported or controlled for; the authors do not elaborate on, or control for, reported differences between the groups on the severity of their injuries, for instance mean differences in the number of days in coma. Hence the apparently greater changes for the experimental versus the control groups may have been caused by premorbid differences between the groups.

The problem of maintenance of micro cognitive therapy gains was specifically addressed by Marks, Parente and Anderson (1986). These authors investigated intensive (2–4 hours per day) memory training using home-based micros, over a sustained period (6–12 months). Their experimental and control groups consisted of 10 head-injured patients, the control group receiving no computer therapy. After cessation of micro-administered treatment, the experimental group was followed up 6–12 months later. Generalization was noted, in that the experimental patients showed significant rises in Wechsler memory quotients (Wechsler, 1945) over the training period ($P<0.05$), and these gains were maintained 6–12 months post-therapy. The results of these two studies (Kerner and Acker, 1985; Marks *et al.*, 1986) suggest that intensive and prolonged micro-based memory treatment may be necessary to sustain the cognitive gains made once training has finished.

Towle, Edmans and Lincoln (1988) examined the effect of roughly 18 sessions of computerized memory therapy over a period of six weeks on eleven patients who had suffered strokes an average of approximately six months previously. The patients all reported memory impairments on a standardized subjective memory questionnaire.

The rationale for the training was one of non-specific stimulation of memory through a range of tasks including word, picture and face recall and recognition as well as several others offered in a game format on BBC computers.

Of five memory tests given (subjective memory questionnaire; recognition memory – words and figures; prose recall – immediate and delayed), none showed a significant change with the exception of immediate prose recall which showed a significant improvement, from a mean of 4 items recalled, to a mean of 5.5. The authors are careful to point out that, as there was no control group, then this single significant change could have occurred for many reasons other than the computer stimulation, for instance a practice or general stimulation effect. They emphasize the need for evaluation of computerized cognitive rehabilitation and do not recommend that this type of therapy be offered routinely to memory disordered patients because of the tiny effects and lack of generalization of such effects. Given the massive drawbacks of A-B designs as mentioned above, their conclusions seem to be appropriate.

Batchelor, Shores, Marosszeky, Sandanam and Lovarini (1988) used a wide variety of commercially available software aimed at rehabilitating 'one or more of the following areas: recent memory (verbal or nonverbal); attention/speed of information processing, higher cognitive functioning' (p. 80). Twenty hours of this therapy administered by computer was compared with twenty hours of such therapy administered manually. Thirty-four severely head-injured patients were alternately allocated to the two groups and neuropsychological testing carried out pre- and post-training. No statistically significant results emerged between groups.

Smart and Richards (1986) described the cognitive rehabilitation software developed at Dundee University for use with head-injured patients, patients experiencing visuospatial deficits, and young children. Their rehabilitation programs include those addressing memory impairment: 'Word Recall' is an adaptive recall program for treating short-term memory deficits, and 'Memory Squares' focuses on visuospatial and memory deficits using recall for combinations of coloured squares. Their preliminary results with head-injured patients suggested that touch-sensitive screens show good acceptance and also solve the problem of the patient forgetting how to respond via the micro. As long as motor tremor is not severe, response areas on the VDU of 5 cm square do not cause response problems.

In reviewing the use of micros in cognitive rehabilitation, Kurlychek and Levin (1987) point to the need for specialized software to be developed (particularly given the limitations of video games), mentioning the 'Cogrehab' programs marketed by Life Science Associates.

'Cogrehab 1' consists of nine programs targeted on visuoperceptual and memory deficits, and 'Cogrehab 3' concentrates on memory exercises for patients functioning at a higher level (Gianutsos and Klitzner, 1981; Gianutsos and Klitzner, 1983). The programs run on Apples, Franklin, Tandy, and IBM-PC micros. The 'Cogrehab 1' memory programs comprise 'Freerec' and 'Triprec' (measure short- and long-term memory using free recall), 'Span' (aimed at retraining short-term memory capacity, and 'Segrec' (suitable for even severely damaged patients, this employs sequential recall on a non-verbal task). Each program costs approximately $30. 'Cogrehab 3' includes 2 memory tasks – 'Wordmem' (training for immediate verbal span, using a random list of words) and 'Pairmem' (training to assist associative verbal learning, using pairs of unrelated words). The recently-available 'Cogrehab 4' from Life Science Associates includes a program ('Attend') which focuses upon attentional deficit using a set of vigilance tasks. These publishers also market a micro version of the Randt Memory Test (Brown, Randt and Osborne, 1983), which might be particularly appropriate for elderly people, and which offers normative and clinical data.

Smith's Cognitive Rehabilitation Series (described by Kurlychek and Levin, 1987) contains many rehabilitation programs including one to assist in compensatory recall and recognition training following memory impairment. Of particular value may be the software which allows the clinician to modify and expand some of the included programs.

The software developed by Bracy (1986) includes memory training routines (marketed through Psychological Software Services). His software runs on Apple, Atari and IBM micros. The 'Foundation II' package (about $300) contains programs designed to assess and exercise attentional and vigilance processes. The 'Memory I and II' packages (approximately $300 each) both contain exercises in spatial and verbal memory functioning. 'Memory I' also includes a sequenced recognition task for short words, and an auditory memory (sequences of tones) task. 'Memory II' contains a visual sequential memory exercise, a paired-associate learning task (graphic figures and digits), and a verbal memory routine which involves categorization and recall.

A particularly elaborate software package is the Einstein Memory Trainer (Einstein Corporation, 1983), which runs on Atari and Commodore C64 micros. The package comprises six programs, run on four disks. Rather than treatment *per se*, the software is aimed at members of the general public who wish to improve their memory. Lesson 1 ('names and faces') teaches associations between facial aspects and peg names to aid recall of 'the names of people you meet'. Lesson 2 ('method of loci') teaches the use of a mental map to locate to-be-remembered information items at familiar locations. Lessons 3, 4 and 5 describe and apply the peg-word memory aid. The final program ('memory mix game') allows the opportunity to practise what has been learnt in the preceding lessons. The Einstein Memory Trainer has potential application to memory-impaired people, although it is too high level and slow/complex in running, in its present form, to be of general relevance to patients with memory deficits.

Although the available software for memory rehabilitation is now expanding quickly, there is still a lack of definite proof regarding the effectiveness of micro therapy. Bracy, Lynch, Sbordone and Berrol (1985), whilst discussing the evolution of micros in cognitive rehabilitation from their initial point as game-playing machines, cautioned against the assumption that micros are bound to be the best way to teach a skill: optimal learning may require a close approximation between training task and real-life task. However, the micro does offer repeated treatment trials without clinician exhaustion or boredom, great flexibility in terms of level of difficulty, and perhaps the less threatening environment of simulation rather than real life. It seems clear that the involvement of micros in memory assessment and rehabilitation is justified from an efficiency viewpoint.

Undoubtedly, micro administration has a number of advantages (see introductory section in this chapter), and the research on cognitive assessment is convincing. For some tasks, micro versions of traditional tests are possible, and the work of Beaumont and French (1987), Moerland *et al.* (1988), Schlichting and Wray (1986), and Acker (1980) has been of value in this respect. However, a micro's features will continue to be under-exploited if research is merely seeking to extend the range of 'conversions' of traditional tests available on a micro. Beaumont and French argued for more 'intelligent' test systems to be designed and developed, and workers in the field should be encouraged to build upon psychological theory regarding cognitive processes, and to involve tasks developed within experimental psychology when designing new cognitive test procedures, rather than mimicking traditional psychometric tests.

Confirmation of the therapeutic effectiveness of micro software may gradually emerge in the light of clinical experience with cognitive rehabilitation programs (e.g. Bracy *et al.*, 1985). However, the question is better addressed by a more rigorous investigation, and the available literature is still thin and often of the 'case study' variety, which presents problems in drawing general conclusions. For example, Finlayson *et al.* (1987) seemed to make extravagant claims for micro retraining, whereas Wood and Fussey (1987) might have been unduly cautious with regard to their findings. The recent study by Sohlberg and Mateer (1987), also attempting to remediate attentional deficits, supported the latter's findings. A number of evaluations of cognitive rehabilitation software are currently underway, including that being carried out in Edinburgh (Gray and Robertson, 1989). Gray and Robertson's early findings add weight to the evidence that specific improvement in attentional processes can be achieved using treatment programs delivered by micro.

The Edinburgh research failed to find an effect of computerized training on unilateral visual neglect (Robertson, Gray *et al.*, 1990), in a randomized controlled trial with six months post-treatment blind follow-up. A parallel, as yet unpublished, study by the same group did however find in a second randomized controlled trial that computerized attentional training did apparently cause differential improvement of the experimental group on WAIS arithmetic and block design as well as on PASAT. Strangely, however, this effect was only apparent at a statistically significant level some six months after treatment ended! Hence the effect must be treated with caution and replication is urgently needed.

A study by Sturm *et al.*, (1983) also found positive effects of attentional training, however, albeit soon after training and not some months afterwards. In an elegant crossover design, they found that training using the 'Vienna Test System' – a range of attention and perceptual speed tasks – produced predictable improvement in a wide range of intellectual functions over the course of training for the treated but not for the control group. These effects were stable for at least four weeks following cessation of training.

Taking the Edinburgh studies, the Sohlberg and Mateer paper and the Sturm *et al.* study, and while acknowledging the existence of negative findings such as those by Ponsford and Kinsella (1988), there seem to be greater grounds for optimism that attentional training by computers may have considerably more promise than either memory or perceptual training.

This conclusion, expanded by Robertson (1990) in a review of computerized cognitive rehabilitation, also applies to some extent to language rehabilitation, where recent as yet unpublished research by Katz and colleagues in the United States suggests significant effects of computerized language training for a range of acquired language disorders. Stachowiak *et al.* (1989) have also reported significant effects of a general computerized language training programme lasting 30 hours on the test performance in an extremely large randomized controlled trial carried out in Germany. Bruce and Howard (1987) also showed how computers could be used effectively to generate phonemic cues in people with naming difficulties.

The cautious optimism about attention and language training does not apply to more generalized attempts to improve cognitive function using computerized training procedures. In one study by Ethier *et al.* (1989), over 100 hours of training on a range of commercially available cognitive rehabilitation software over a period of six months failed to produce significant improvements even on the training programmes themselves, suggesting that these subjects were exposed to a uniquely fruitless and time-consuming experience.

Skinner and Trachtman (1985) described the development of a 'colouring book' program for use in cognitive rehabilitation. The program runs on IBM-compatible PCs, offering a simulation of a child's colouring book. The program is 'mouse' controlled for ease of menu option choice and error correction. The latter study employed a 'mouse' (hand-operated control for pointing to and selecting options displayed on the micro's screen) as response device because of its ease of use. Few reports have appeared which have investigated the important area of type of response device and patient performance and acceptability. If at all possible patient response through a micro's standard keyboard should be avoided – too much information-processing is required of the patient and the probability of an erroneous entry is high. Response method is obviously very relevant for some patients, particularly those with physical impairments or significant cognitive deficit. A number of appropriate response methods have been devised and investigated. For example, Norris, *et al.*, (1985) described the design and use of a customized response board for the Commodore PET. Beaumont (1985) compared the speed of response obtained from a standard QWERTY keyboard, numeric keypad, light pen, and touch-sensitive screen. His results indicated that the quickest response times were obtained using the touch screen, followed by the keypad, keyboard, and light pen. The latter appeared slowest due to hardware 'lag', although these response devices can also be somewhat unwieldy to use.

Smart and Richards (1986) reported on the use of touch-sensitive screens in rehabilitation. They noted that a membrane touch screen (screen placed in front of the monitor) has the drawbacks of reducing and diffusing light from the VDU, lowering clarity, and a vulnerability to accidental damage. The latter susceptibility mitigates against its use with patients, whereas the 'contact' touch screen does not suffer this disadvantage. However, a patient user of a contact screen might be disconcerted by the machine's functioning, given that contact with the screen is not necessary (only close proximity) to register a response. Smart and Richards recommended contact touch screens for rehabilitation work, particularly as commercially available versions of these are now inexpensive.

## SUMMARY AND FUTURE DEVELOPMENTS

Micros offer a number of advantages in cognitive assessment and treatment, including cost/time-saving, flexibility, provision of controlled conditions, timed responses, patient acceptability, and ease of data analysis. They present relatively few potential disadvantages. Micros may be employed to test cognitive functions, assess the effectiveness of a therapeutic intervention, or may be used in providing the treatment for cognitive dysfunction. A small number of cognitive assessment 'batteries' have been developed over the last few years (e.g. Acker, 1980; Moerland *et al.*, 1986), some of which have concentrated upon 'translating', or producing analogues of, psychometric tests (e.g. Beaumont and French, 1987). Most researchers, however, have concentrated upon developing a single micro-based cognitive task, and an increasing range of these is now available.

It seems clear that the greatest contribution to clinical practice will be made if investigators use the particular features of their micro to develop cognitive assessment tasks which relate as directly as possible to psychological theory by drawing upon tasks employed in experimental psychology; for example, by explaining in detail memory performance via microcomputer task which offer very sensitive response timing routines.

This capacity for millisecond timing offers a role for micros in detecting, and describing, the often subtle cognitive changes associated with medication effects; this can be very valuable when undertaking therapeutic trials of drugs. Available guidance on the important elements involved in cognitive retraining (Kurlycheck and Levin, 1987) serve to emphasize the compatibility with micro-delivered therapy. Evidence is beginning to emerge which supports the effectiveness of micro-based cognitive treatment, particularly where attentional deficits are being addressed.

Some useful initial work on the various types of patient response device which might be employed in conjunction with micro-based cognitive tasks has also been carried out, with contact touch screens being recommended.

With regard to future developments, good demonstrations of the therapeutic benefits associated with micro memory treatment programs are now available, though generalization and persistence of gains remains to be adequately proven. The parameters of duration and intensity of memory therapy via micro also need to be addressed. We should expect to see an increase in the amount and range of specialized software available to use in the field of cognitive deficit and, as mentioned above, test development will probably draw more upon the theoretical underpinnings of cognitive psychology. Research is needed to identify predictive factors in micro-based therapy – which tasks and software are most appropriate for particular deficits, and how do other clinical and intrapersonal factors affect outcome. In the future there will also be a move towards increasing the flexibility of software, allowing clinicians to modify programs to suit their needs. Finally, there will be the inevitable development over time of normative standards and clinical data.

## REFERENCES

Acker, W. (1980) In Support of Microcomputer-Based Automated Testing: A Description of the Maudsley Automated Psychological Screening Tests. *British Journal of Alcoholism and Addiction,* **15**, 144–47.

Algarabel, S. (1983) MEMORIA: A Computer Program for Experimental Control of Verbal Learning and Memory Experiments with the Apple II Microcomputer. Behaviour Research Methods and Instrumentation, **15**, 394.

Angle, H.B., Hay, L.R., Hay, W.M. and Ellinwood, E.H. (1977) Computer-Aided Interviewing in Comprehensive Behavioural Assessment. *Behaviour Therapy,* **8**. 747–54.

Batchelor, J, Shore, E, Marosszeky, J, Sandanam, J, and Lovarini, M. (1988) Cognitive rehabilitation of severely closed-head-injured patients using computer-assisted and noncomputerised treatment techniques. *Journal of Head Trauma Rehabilitation* **3**, 78–85.

Benton, A.L. (1974) *The Revised Visual Retention Test* (4th edn). New York: Psychological Corporation.

Beaumont, J.G. (1985) Speed of Response Using Keyboard and Screen-Based Microcomputer Response Media. *International Journal of Man-Machine Studies,* **23**, 61–70.

Beaumont, J.G. and French, C.C. (1987) Clinical Field Study of Eight Automated Psychometric Procedures: The Leicester/DHSS Project. *International Journal of Man-Machine Studies,* **26**, 661–82.

Bracy, O.L. (1986) *Programs For Cognitive Rehabilitation.* Psychological Software Services, Indianapolis

Bracy, O., Lynch, W., Sbordone, R. and Berrol, S. (1985) Cognitive Retraining through Computers: Fact or Fad? *Cognitive Rehabilitation,* **3**, 10–23.

Brown, E.R., Randt, C.T. and Osborne, D.P. Jnr, (1983) Assessment of memory disturbances in aging. In *Aging: Aging Brain and Ergot Alkaloids,* ed. Agnoli *et al.*, Raven Press, New York, **23** pp. 131–7:

Bruce, C. and Howard, D. (1987) Computer-generated phonemic cues: an effective aid for naming in aphasia. *British Journal of Disorders of Communication* **22**, 191–201.

Calistri, R.J. and Kallman, H.J. (1986) DRT/***: Programs to Administer and Score the Diagnostic Rhyme Test. *Behaviour Research Methods, Instruments, and Computers,* **18**, 57–8.

Carr, A.C., Ghosh, A. and Ancill, R.J. (1983) Can a Computer Take a Psychiatric History? *Psychological Medicine,* **13**, 151–8.

Cliffe, M.J. (1985) Microcomputer Implementation of an Idiographic Psychological Instrument. *International Journal of Man-Machine Studies,* **23**, 89–96.

Dahlstrom, W.G., Welsh, G.S. and Dahlstrom, L.E. (1975) *An MMPI Handbook* (vol. 1, Clinical Interpretation, Revised Edn) University of Minnesota Press: Minneapolis.

De Mita, M.A., Johnson, J.H. and Hansen, K.E. (1981) The Validity of a Computerized Visual Searching Task as an Indicator of Brain Damage. *Behaviour Research Methods and Instrumentation,* **13**, 592–4.

Einstein Corporation (1983) *The Einstein Memory Trainer: User Guide.* Los Angeles, California.

Ethier, M. Braun, C. and Baribeau, J. (1989) Computer-dispensed cognitive-perceptual training of closed-head-injury patients after spontaneous recovery. Study 1, speeded tasks. *Canadian Journal of Rehabilitation* **2**, 223–33.

Finlayson, M.A.J., Alfano, D.P. and Sullivan, J.F. (1987) A Neuro-psychological Approach to Cognitive Remediation: Microcomputer Applications. *Canadian Psychology,* **28**, 181–90.

Gedye, J.L. and Miller, E. (1970) Developments in Automated Testing Systems. In P. Mittler (Ed), *The Psychological Assessment of Mental and Physical Handicaps.* Methuen and Co, London, pp. 735–60.

Gianutsos, R. (1983) *COGREHAB VOLUME III: Therapeutic Memory Exercises for Independent Use.* Life Science Associates, New York.

Gianutsos, R. and Klitzner, C. (1981) *Computer Programs for Cognitive Rehabilitation: Personal Computing for Survivors of Brain Injury.* Proceedings of John Hopkins First National Search for Applications with Personal Computing to Aid the Handicapped.

Gianutsos, R. and Klitzner, C. (1983) *COGREHAB VOL I: Perceptual and Memory Programs.* Life Science Associates, New York.

Gray, J.M. and Robertson, I. (1989) Remediation of Attentional Difficulties Following Brain Injury: Three Experimental Single Case Studies. *Brain Injury,* **3**, 163–70.

Holden, U.P. and Woods, R.T. (1982) *Reality Orientation: Psychological Approaches to the Confused Elderly.* Churchill Livingstone, London.

Johnson, R. and Garvie, C. (1985) The BBC Microcomputer for Therapy of Intellectual Impairment following Acquired Brain Damage. *Occupational Therapy,* February 1985, 46–8.

Kerner, M.J. and Acker, M. (1985) Computer Delivery of Memory Retraining with Head-Injured Patients. *Cognitive Rehabilitation,* **3**, 26–31.

Kurlychek, R.T. and Levin, W. (1987) Computers in the Cognitive

Rehabilitation of Brain-Injured Persons. *CRC Critical Reviews in Medical Informatics*, **1**, 241–57.

Lezak, M.D. (1983) *Neuropsychological Assessment* (second ed). Oxford University Press.

Lucas, R.W. (1977) A Study of Patients' Attitudes to Computer Interrogation. *International Journal of Man-Machine Studies*, **9** 69–86.

Marks, C., Parente, F. and Anderson, J. (1986) Retention of Gains in Outpatient Cognitive Rehabilitation Therapy. *Cognitive Rehabilitation*, 4, 20–3.

Moerland, M.C., Alderkamp, A.P. and De Alpherts, W.C.J. (1986) A Neuropsychological Test Battery for the Apple II-e. *International Journal of Man-Machine Studies*, **25**, 453–67.

Moffat, N J. (1989) *Use of BBC Micro with Demented Patients*. Personal Communication.

Money, J.A. (1976) *A Standardized Road Map Test of Direction Sense: Manual.* Academic Therapy Publications, Chicago.

Morris, R.G. (1985) Automated Clinical Assessment. In F.N. Watts (ed): *New Developments in Clinical Psychology*, BPS/Wiley.

Mulhall, D.J. (1980) *Manual for the Personal Questionnaire Rapid Scaling Technique.* NFER Publishing Co., Windsor.

Nelson, T.O. and Narens, L. (1980) Norms of 300 general-information questions: accuracy of recall, latency of recall, and feeling-of-knowing ratings. *Journal of Verbal Learning and Verbal Behaviour*, **19**, 338–68.

Norris, D., Skilbeck, C.E., Haywood, A.E and Torpy, D. (1985) *Microcomputer in Clinical Practice.* John Wiley.

Ponsford, J. and Kinsella, G. (1988) Evaluation of a remedial programme for attentional deficits following closed head injury. *Journal of Clinical and Experimental Neuropsychology* **10**, 693–708.

Randt, C.T., Brown, E.R., and Osborne, D.P. (1980) A Memory Test for Longitudinal Measurement of Mild to Moderate Deficiencies. *Clinical Neuropsychology*, **2**, 184–94.

Raven, J.C. (1983) *Standard Progressive Matrices: Manual.* H.K. Lewis and Co., London.

Reitan, R. M. (1979) *Neuropsychology and Rehabilitation*. University of Tucson.

Robertson. I. (1990) Does computerised cognitive rehabilitation work? A review. *Aphasiology*, **4**, 381–405.

Robertson, I. Gray, J. Pentland, B. and Waite, L. (1990) A randomised controlled trial of computer-based cognitive rehabilitation for unilateral left visual neglect. *Archives of Physical Medicine and Rehabilitation*, **71**, 663–8.

Ryan, E.D. (1986) Memory for Goblins: A computer Game for Assessing and Training Working Memory Skill. *Clinical Gerontologist*, **6**, 64–7.

Sanders, R. L. (1985) Computer-Administered Individualised Psychological Testing: The Feasibility Study. *International Journal of Man-Machine Studies*, **23**, 197–213.

Schlichting, C. and Wray, D. (1986) COGNITION: A Program for the Presentation of Several Tests of Cognitive Function using the Hewlett – Packard 85 Computer. *Behaviour Research Methods Instruments, and Computers*, **18**, 65.

Shimamura, A.P., Landwehr, R.F. and Nelson, T.O. (1981) FACT-RETRIEVAL: A Programme for Assessing Someone's Recall of general information facts, feeling-of-knowing-judgements for non-recalled facts, and recognition of non-recalled facts. *Behaviour Research Methods and Instrumentation*, **13**, 691–2.

Skilbeck, C.E. (1989) *An Information-Processing Approach to Cognitive Recovery Following Head Injury*. Unpublished PhD Thesis.

Skilbeck, C.E. and Woods, R.T. (1980) The Factorial Structure of the Wechsler Memory Scale: Samples of Neurological and Psychogeriatric patients. *Journal of Clinical Neuropsychology*, **2**, 293–300.

Skinner, A.D. and Trachtman, L.H. (1985) Brief or New: Use of a Computer Program (PC Colouring Book) in Cognitive Rehabilitation. *American Journal of Occupational Therapy*, **39**, 470–2.

Slack, W.V. and Slack, C.W. (1977) Talking to a Computer about emotional problems: A Comparative Study. *Psychotherapy: Theory, Research and Practice*, **14**, 156–64.

Smart, S. and Richards, D. (1986) The Use of Touch Sensitive Screens in Rehabilitation Therapy. *Occupational Therapy*, October, 335–8.

Sohlberg, M. and Mateer, A. (1987) Effectiveness of an attention-training programme. *Journal of Clinical and Experimental Neuropsychology*, **9**, 117–30.

Space, L. G. (1981) The Computer as Psychometrician. *Behaviour Research Methods and Instrumentation*, **13**, 595–606.

Stachowiak, F. Geilffuss, J. Helgeson, H. Lobin, U. Schadler, G. Seggewies, G. and Willke, A. (in press) *Effekte der computerunterstützten Sprachtherapie*. Tagungsbericht, Symposium 'Computer helfen heilen'. Kliniken Schmieder, Gailingen-Allensbach, 1989. Bonn: Kuratorium ZNS, Humboldtstrasse 30, 53 Bonn 1, Federal Republic of Germany.

Sternberg, S. (1969) Memory Scanning: Mental Processes Revealed by Reaction Time Experiments. *American Scientist*, **4**, 421–57.

Sturm, W. Dahmen, W. Hartje, W. and Wilmes, K. (1983) Ergebnisse eines Trainingsprogramms zur Verbesserung der visuellen Auffassungsshnelligkeit und Konzentrationsfähigkeit bei Hirngeschädigten. *Archive für Psychiatre und Nervenkrankenheiten* **233**, 9–22.

Towle O., Edmans, J.A. and Lincoln, N.B. (1988) Use of computer-presented games with memory-impaired stroke patients. *Clinical Rehabilitation* 2 303–7.

van Zomeren, A.H. and Deelman, B.G. (1978) Long-Term Recovery of Visual Reaction Time After Closed Head Injury. *Journal of Neurology, Neurosurgery and Psychiatry*, **41**, 452–5.

Wechsler, D. (1945) *Wechsler Memory Scale: Manual* New York: The Psychological Corporation.

Wechsler, D. (1987) *Wechsler Adult Intelligence Scale – Revised*. New York: The Psychological Corporation.

Wood, R.L. and Fussey, I. (1987) Computer-Based Cognitive Retraining: A Controlled Study. *International Journal of Disability Studies*, **9**, 149–153.

## REFERENCE NOTE

*Journal of Cognitive Rehabilitation*, Odie L. Bracy (Ed), 6555 Carrollton Ave., Indianapolis, IN 46220, USA.

1. Computer Version of Randt Memory Test.
2. Computer Programme for Cognitive Rehabilitation by R. Gianutsos and others. Both are obtainable from:

Life Science Associates, One Fenimore Road, Bayport, NY 11705, USA.

# Chapter 7

# The psychopharmacology of human memory disorders

## MICHAEL D. KOPELMAN

## THE NEUROPSYCHOLOGY AND NEUROCHEMISTRY OF MEMORY DISORDERS

### The amnesic (Korsakoff) syndrome

Despite continuing controversy regarding the explanation of the memory deficit(s) in the organic amnesic syndrome, there is reasonable agreement in the description of its characteristic features. Performance at span tests is preserved (Zangwill, 1946; Drachman and Arbitt, 1966), and some studies, but not all, find absolute or relative preservation of verbal 'short-term' forgetting (Baddeley and Warrington, 1970; Kopelman, 1985; but contrast Butters and Cermak, 1980). There is a severe impairment in performance at 'explicit' learning tests, but procedural memory, the response to priming, and many well-rehearsed aspects of semantic memory, remain intact (e.g. Warrington and Weiskrantz, 1970; Brooks and Baddeley, 1976; Graf Squire and Mandler, 1984). Moreover, once learning has been established (e.g. by manipulating the exposure times of material to be learned), the rate of 'long-term' forgetting is usually normal (Huppert and Piercy, 1978; Kopelman 1985; Baddeley, Harris, Sunderland Watts and Wilson, 1987). In addition, there is commonly a retrograde component to the memory loss, which encompasses the recall both of auto-biographical incidents and of 'personal semantic' facts about the subject's past (Kopelman, Wilson and Baddeley, 1989). This retrograde component is very variable in its extensiveness: in head injury, it is often brief and well correlated with the length of post-traumatic amnesia (Russell and Smith, 1961), whereas in the Korsakoff syndrome, it is extensive and poorly correlated with the severity of anterograde amnesia (Shimamura and Squire, 1986; Kopelman, 1989).

### Alzheimer-type dementia

In Alzheimer-type dementia, there is the same severe impairment in learning 'explicit' material, but the memory deficits appear to be more extensive than in the organic amnesic syndrome (for review, see Morris and Kopelman, 1986; Huppert, 1989). There is substantial impairment at tests of primary or working memory, whether measured in terms of span test performance (Kaszniak, Garron and Fox, 1979; Morris, 1984; Kopelman, 1985), the recency component of free recall (although the precise measurement and interpretation of this is debated: Wilson, Bacon, Fox, and Kaszniak, 1983; Martin, Brouwers, Cox and Fedio, 1985; Spinnler, Della Sala, Bandera and Baddeley, 1988), and verbal and non-verbal 'short-term' forgetting (Corkin, 1982; Kopelman, 1985; Morris, 1986; Sullivan, Corkin and Growdon, 1986; Dannenbaum, Parkinson and Inman, 1988). There have been relatively few studies of procedural memory, some studies indicating that it is preserved (Eslinger and Damasio, 1986; Knopman and Nissen, 1987) and others indicating impairment (Grober, 1985). Similarly, there are studies which find a preserved response to priming (Miller, 1975; Morris, Wheatley and Britton 1983), and others which find impaired priming (Shimamura, Salmon and Squire, 1987). Semantic memory is much more severely impaired than in the Korsakoff syndrome, especially on naming and verbal fluency tasks (Huff, Corkin and Growdon 1986; Ober et al., 1986; Hart Smith and Swash, 1988), although it is interesting to note that the ability to make use of meaning in memory tasks appears well preserved in the early stages of the disorder (Nebes, Martin and Horn, 1984; Kopelman, 1986a). As in the organic amnesic syndrome, the rate of 'long-term' forgetting appears to be normal once learning has been accomplished (Kopelman, 1985; Becker *et al.*, 1987); and there is an extensive retrograde loss with a 'gentle' temporal gradient, less steep than that seen in the Korsakoff syndrome (Sagar *et al.*, 1988; Kopelman *et al.*, 1989).

## Huntington's disease

Huntington's disease is the only other type of dementia in which the pattern of memory impairment has been studied in detail. In this disorder, there is a progressive onset of anterograde and retrograde memory impairment (Aminoff *et al.* 1975; Albert, Butters and Brandt, 1981). In the more advanced stages of the disorder Huntington patients show a severe 'explicit' memory impairment, similar to that seen in Korsakoff and Alzheimer patients, but they tend to produce fewer intrusion errors than do the other two groups (Butters *et al.*, 1987). They also show severe impairment at tests of 'short-term' forgetting (Meudell Butters and Montgomery, 1978; Butters and Cermak, 1980) and at procedural memory (Marton *et al.*, 1984), but the response to verbal priming is intact (Shimamura *et al.*, 1987). Performance of verbal fluency tasks is impaired whereas confrontation naming is intact (Butters *et al.*, 1987), possibly indicating that those aspects of semantic memory are impaired which are critically dependent upon frontal lobe function. Once learning has been accomplished, the rate of 'long-term' forgetting is normal (Martone, Butters and Trauner, 1986); and there is an extensive retrograde impairment, in which Butters and his colleagues fail to find any evidence of a temporal gradient (Albert *et al.*, 1981; Beatty, Salmon and Butters; 1988).

## Neurochemistry of these disorders

In the alcoholic Korsakoff syndrome, there is evidence that acetylcholine, GABA, glutamate and aspartate (all putative neurotransmitters) may show reduced turnover or synthesis, as a result of thiamine depletion (Witt, 1985). There is also evidence that cholinergic neurones may be depleted (Arendt *et al.*, 1983), and that noradrenergic and serotinergic pathways may be implicated (McEntee, Mair and Langlais, 1984; Witt, 1985). In Alzheimer's disease, there is very substantial evidence that there is cortical and subcortical cholinergic depletion (Rossor, Iversen and Reynolds, 1984; Kopelman, 1986b). There is also evidence of GABA and noradrenergic depletion (Rossor, Garrett and Johnson, 1982; Rossor *et al.*, 1984) as well as involvement of many other pututative neurotransmitters (Rossor and Iversen, 1986; Kopelman, 1986b). In Huntington's disease, there is depletion of GABA in the striatum and substantia nigra, but findings with respect to other neurotransmitters are equivocal (Perry, Hansten and Kloster, 1973; Thomlinson and Corsellis, 1984). In particular, there does not appear to be any depletion of subcortical cholinergic neurones (Arendt *et al.*, 1983; Clark, Parhad, and Folstein, 1983).

There is substantial evidence that cholinergic antagonist drugs (cholinergic 'blockers') impair memory in healthy subjects providing a 'model' for the effect of cholinergic depletion and suggesting the possible role of cholinergic 'replacement' in memory remediation. There is also considerable evidence that benzodiazepines produce memory impairment but, paradoxically, these drugs are thought to *potentiate* the actions of the GABA system. There is also evidence that noradrenergic-antagonizing drugs may impair memory, but this is much more equivocal. The next section will review the action of these drugs on the kinds of memory processes discussed above. Particular attention will be paid to the cholinergic system, because this has been the most fully investigated.

STUDIES OF THE EFFECTS OF AGENTS MODULATING NEURO-
TRANSMITTER SYSTEMS IN HEALTHY SUBJECTS

### Studies of cholinergic blockers

The difficulties of conducting this type of study have been discussed elsewhere (Kopelman, 1986b; Kopelman and Corn, 1988). Various studies have been conducted in healthy subjects, which have investigated the effect of the cholinergic blocker, hyoscine/scopolamine, upon aspects of attention and memory, respectively. It should be noted that hyoscine exerts its predominant effects upon the so-called muscarinic receptors in the brain but that, at higher doses, it also antagonizes nicotine receptors (Weiner, 1980) and, indeed, nicotine has been shown to reverse some of its effects (Wesnes and Revell, 1984).

In general, there are variable results on tests of attention and information processing but many studies reveal impairment. It appears that dual-channel tasks (Drachman, Noffsinger and Sahakian, 1980; Dunne and Hartley, 1985) and vigilance tasks conducted over an extended period (Wesnes and Warburton, 1983, 1984) are particularly sensitive to the effect of cholinergic blockade. There appears to be quite a striking dose-response effect, and this is particularly well illustrated in studies by Safer and Allen (1971), Nuotto (1983), Wesnes and Warburton (1984), and Parrott (1986).

Dunne and Hartley (1985) argued that hyoscine can disrupt attentional processes without affecting over-all memory performance. Using a dichotic listening procedure, they instructed subjects to attend to one or other channel whilst a 20-word list was presented (10 words per channel). Administration of hyoscine resulted in a reduction in (immediate and delayed) recall from the attended channel, and no significant effect upon total recall. On recognition testing, over-all performance was also unaffected by the drug, although in this case there was no evidence of a drug x attention interaction. Against that point of view, Dunne and Hartley (1986) failed to obtain an over-all impairment of performance on a target detection task in a later study. Moreover, various studies have reported that hyoscine can produce amnesic deficits at doses which do not impair performance at tests of attention and vigilance (Crow and Grove-White, 1973; Crow, Grove-White, and Ross, 1975; Caine and Weingartner, *et al.*, 1981; Sunderland, Tariot and Cohen, 1987; Kopelman and Corn, 1988); whilst other studies have found fairly uniform impairments across different types of test (Parrott, 1986; Wesnes, Simpson and Kidd, 1988).

There are many studies which have found that cholinergic blockade produces an impairment of explicit memory, whilst performance at span tests or the recency component of free recall remains unaffected (e.g. Crow and Grove-White, 1973; Drachman and Leavitt, 1974; Frith, Richardson and Samuel, 1984; Kopelman and Corn, 1988). Two recent studies have included Alzheimer and Parkinson patients, respectively, demonstrating that these groups show lower dose thresholds for the manifestation of 'explicit' memory impairment (Dubois, Danze and Pillon, 1987; Sunderland *et al.*, 1987). Only the more recent studies have examined the pattern of memory deficits in a detailed fashion, similar to that employed in the studies of patient groups discussed above (Caine *et al.*, 1981; Beatty, Butters and Janowsky, 1986; Nissen, Knopman and Schacter, 1987; Kopelman and Corn, 1988).

Caine *et al.* (1981) found impairment on verbal and nonverbal recall tests of explicit memory as well as impairment on a version of the Brown-Peterson ('short-term' forgetting) task, in a small group of patients (Brown, 1958; Peterson and Peterson, 1959). Caine *et al.* also showed that the verbal recall impairment could, apparently, be mitigated by providing semantic or acoustic retrieval cues; and it is possible that this finding may have reflected a preserved priming phenomenon. (The experimental details are not clear regarding this point). Beatty *et al.* (1986) demonstrated impaired verbal memory, and impairment at a version of the Brown-Peterson task in which the precise form of the distractor task was varied. Verbal fluency (semantic retrieval) was intact. These authors argued that a different pattern of errors was obtained in cholinergic blockade from that seen in Alzheimer dementia, but their data on this point were not very convincing. Nissen *et al.* (1987) showed impairment on verbal recall and recognition tests with intact ability at a procedural memory task (serial reaction time) and at two semantic retrieval tasks. Results on a repetition priming task were equivocal.

Kopelman and Corn (1988) conducted a study in 70 subjects using tests identical or closely similar to those which had previously been used in Alzheimer and Korsakoff patients. It was found that cholinergic blockade did not have a significant effect upon the more passive aspects of working memory, namely span tests and a measure of verbal, short-term forgetting (the Brown-Peterson test). In this, it resembled the Korsakoff syndrome and contrasted with the marked deficits seen in Alzheimer-type dementia. On the other hand, cholinergic blockade did produce impairment at a visuo-spatial, short-term forgetting test, and at a verbal test (Brown-Peterson) in which the distractor task was made more difficult. On tests of secondary memory, cholinergic blockade produced a pattern similar to that seen in the anterograde amnesia of Korsakoff and many Alzheimer patients; namely, a pronounced impairment in learning verbal and visuo-spatial material, a normal forgetting rate once learning had been accomplished, and relative preservation of the response to priming and of procedural memory. However, cholinergic blockade did not produce a retrograde amnesia, nor did it affect the recall of temporal context or of long-established semantic knowledge. A significant effect was also produced upon a measure of subjective arousal and on one of three 'attention' tests which were employed; but co-varying for the latter had negligible effect upon the pattern of performance on the memory tests. Kopelman and Corn (1988) concluded that cholinergic blockade produced a pattern of anterograde amnesia consistent with that seen in the Korsakoff syndrome and many Alzheimer patients, but that it did not mimic the extensive retrograde loss seen in both disorders, nor the severe impairment of primary or working memory which occurs in Alzheimer-type dementia.

## Studies of benzodiazepines

The effects of benzodiazepines on memory have been excellently reviewed by Curran (1986). As in the case of hyoscine/ scopolamine, the amnesia induced by these drugs has a very practical advantage when they are used as an anaesthetic premedication agent (cf. O'Boyle, Barry and Fox, 1987). As in studies of cholinergic blockers, span tasks are usually unaffected (e.g. Brown, Lewis and Brown, 1982; Curran, Schiwy and Lader 1987), and the recency component of free recall is also spared in most studies (e.g. Ghoneim and Mewalt, 1975). Administered before learning, these drugs produce an anterograde impairment in 'explicit' memory (e.g. Ghoneim and Mewaldt, 1975, 1977; Curran *et al.*, 1987), sensitive to both recall and recognition testing (Brown *et al.*, 1982) and very similar to that produced by hyoscine/scopolamine (Frith *et al.*, 1984), except that it is reversed by a benzodiazepine antagonist (Dorow, Berenberg and Duka,

1987) but not by a cholinergic agent (Ghoneim and Mewaldt, 1977). Tasks involving verbal material are more consistently affected than those involving pictorial material (Curran, 1986). Once learning has been accomplished, the rate of forgetting is normal (Brown, Brown and Bowes, 1983), and these drugs do not produce any retrograde deficit (Ghoneim and Mewaldt, 1975, 1977), and may even facilitate the recall of material learned immediately before drug administration (Brown *et al.*, 1982; Ghoneim, Mewaldt and Heinrichs, 1984). Retrieval from semantic memory is slowed by these drugs (Brown *et al.*, 1983; Ghoneim *et al.*, 1984), but the over-all level of performance is not significantly affected (Brown *et al.*, 1983). Curran (1986) concludes that sedation contributes to, but probably does not completely account for, the amnesic effects of benzodiazepines; and Brown *et al.* (1982) and Lister and Weingartner (1987) have pointed to the similarity between the anterograde amnesia they produce and that of the alcoholic Korsakoff syndrome.

### Studies of drugs modulating the adrenergic system

There have also been a number of studies examining the effect of adrenergic agents upon memory and, in particular, investigating vasopressin which may modulate noradrenergic neuro-transmission (De Wied and van Ree, 1982). Much of this work derives from De Wied's animal studies, but there is considerable controversy concerning whether vasopressin exerts its primary effect upon memory *per se* or upon arousal and mood (Gash and Thomas, 1983; Sahgal, 1984; De Wied, 1984). For example, Weingartner, Golp and Ballenger, (1981) and Millar, Jeffcoate and Walder (1987) have suggested that vasopressin enhances explicit memory in healthy subjects without affecting semantic memory, whereas Snel, Taylor and Wegman (1987) postulated an effect on 'tonic attentional processes' rather than memory storage or retrieval. Similarly, Frith *et al.* (1985) argued that low doses of clonidine would inhibit noradrenaline release, and these authors found impairment in healthy subjects on a paired-associate learning task, but not on span tests or a semantic memory task (sentence verification). On the other hand, Clark, Geffen and Geffen (1986) found that the most striking effects were on subjective arousal, and that there was significant impairment at both focused and divided attention tasks.

## Clinical trials of 'replacement' therapy in amnesic or dementing patients

Traditional approaches to the pharmacotherapy of memory disorders involved the administration of vasodilator substances (e.g. hydrogenated ergot alkaloids such as 'hydergine'), central nervous system stimulants, hyper-baric oxygen, high potency vitamin preparations, or ribo-nucleic acid to elderly or demented patients. Although some success was claimed in some studies, the over-all results of such trials have been very disappointing (for review, Whitehouse, 1981; Kopelman and Lishman, 1986). More recent studies have focused attention upon attempting to manipulate the neurotransmitter systems considered above.

### Cholinergic agents

Trials of cholinergic 'replacement' therapy have involved the administration of oral choline or lecithin (precursors of acetylcholine), or the infusion of the anti-cholinesterase, physostigmine (which inhibits the breakdown of acetylcholine) or, occasionally, of dimethylaminoethanol or arecoline (a cholinomimetic which acts directly on cholinergic receptors). More recently, there have been trials of RS-86, oral physostigmine, tetra-hydro-aminoacridine (THA), various drug combinations, and nicotine.

The earliest trials of cholinergic agents in amnesic or dementing patients occurred in the late 1970s, and there were initially a few promising findings (e.g. Peters and Levin, 1977). However, reports soon began to appear of negative or negligible results when these substances were administered to Alzheimer patients (e.g. Boyd, and Graham-White, *et al.*, 1977; Etienne, Cauthier and Johnson, 1978; Smith, Swash and Exton-Smith, 1978; Signoret *et al.*, 1978). By the time Bartus, Dean and Beer (1982) published their review of the trials in Alzheimer-type dementia, they were able to report that of seventeen trials using cholinergic precursors (choline or lecithin), ten reported no effect, six reported non-significant trends towards improved cognitive performance, and only one study claimed statistically significant gains. Further trials reported in Johns, Greenwald and Mohs *et al.*, (1983) and Hollander, Mohs and Davis (1986) were equally disappointing. Similarly, a careful study of prolonged (six months') lecithin administration failed to find any over-all benefit of the drug (Little, Levy, Chauqui-Kidd and Hand, 1985), a result which has recently been replicated (Heyman, Schmechel, Wilkinson *et al.*, 1987). Two trials of the muscarinic agonist, RS-86, also failed to show any significant benefit relative to placebo in Alzheimer patients (Bruno, Mohr and Gillespie *et al.*, 1986; Hollander *et al.*, 1987), although one of the studies claimed that there was a 'clinically meaningful' improvement in six out of twelve patients (Hollander *et al.*, 1987). Moreover, the direct infusion of a cholinergic agonist, bethamecol, into the cerebrospinal fluid by way of a cannula into the brain's ventricular system has been equally unsuccessful (Penn *et al.*, 1988; Whitehouse, 1988).

Trials employing intravenous physostigmine or oral THA have appeared to be somewhat more successful. Johns *et al.* (1983) suggested that improvement was likeliest when the dose was titrated in order to identify the optimum dose for each individual subject, and when recognition rather than recall tests were employed. Both these substances are anticholinesterases, preventing the breakdown of acetylcholine, and Johns *et al.* pointed out that these substances differ from choline and lecithin in not requiring intact presynaptic neurons (in which acetylcholine synthesis occurs) in order to achieve their effect. They suggested that this may account for the greater promise of these substances in the trials of replacement therapy to date.

Table 7.1 summarizes the results in trials of physostigmine (including both oral and intravenous studies) and of the (longer acting) THA. It will be seen that in two of the five studies for which Johns *et al.* had claimed some success (those by Smith and Swash, 1979, and Sullivan *et al.*, 1982) the evidence was pretty unconvincing. In general, these trials have tended to produce statistically significant but small benefits, and it is interesting that, even when cognitive

**Table 7.1** Clinical studies of anticholinesterases (Physostigmine unless stated)

| Authors | Dose/Delay till testing | Tests/Ratings | Modality of stimulus | Result |
|---|---|---|---|---|
| Peters and Levin (1979) | 0.005–0.15 mg/kg S/C 20 min (N=3) | Selective reminding test (3 subjects only) | A | No significant effect (but some improvement when given with lecithin) |
| Smith and Swash (1979) | 1 mg S/C 15 min–1 h (N=1) | Various including free recall, object recognition, verbal fluency | A+V | No significant effect (except reduced intrusion errors) |
| Ashford et al. (1981) | 0.5 mg I/V 20 min (N=6) | Selective reminding test Benton Visual Retention tests | A V | No significant effect No significant effect |
| Christie et al. (1981) | 0.25–1 mg I/V; 15 min–1 h (N=11) | Picture recognition test | V | Significant improvement after 15-min infusion at optimal dose. Otherwise NS |
| Davis and Mohs (1982) | 0.125–0.5 mg I/V; 10 min (N–10) | Picture recognition ('more demented') Word recognition ('less demented') Digit span, famous faces | V A A,V | Significant improvement Significant improvement No significant effect |
| Sullivan et al. (1982) | 0.25–0.5 mg I/V; 15 min– 1 h 15 min (N=12) | Verbal and non-verbal PAL* Brown-Peterson | ?A,V A | No reliable improvement No reliable improvement |
| Jotkowitz (1983) | 12–15 mg 0 daily (N=10) | Clinical dementia scale and memory and orientation test | ?A | No significant effect |
| Thal et al. (1983) | lecithin + oral physost. after dose titration (N=8) | Selective reminding test | A | Significant improvement in recall amongst subgroup of 6 cases |

**Table 7.1 cont.**

| Authors | Dose/Delay till testing | Tests/Ratings | Modality of stimulus | Result |
|---|---|---|---|---|
| Davis et al. (1983) | 0.25–1 mg 0 × 2 h (N=4) | Picture recognition | V | Slight improvement in 3 cases |
| Muramato et al. (1979, 1984) | Various doses and adminstr. Testing up to 180 min (N=6) | Selective reminding Bender Gestalt copying | A V | Sig. improvement in 1 cases Sig. improvement in 3 cases Trend improvement in 1 case |
| Mohs et al. (1985) | 0.5–2 mg 0×2 h (N=12) | Alzheimer's disease Assessment: behaviour and cognition | ? | No significant effect |
| Beller et al. (1985) | Graduated dose up to 2 mg 0 every 2 h (N=8) | Selective reminding | A | Statistically sig. but small improvements in 6s |
| Blackwood and Christie (1986) | 0.75 mg infused I/V per half hour 30–45 min (N=11) | Picture recognition test | V | Significant improvement (P300 unchanged) |
| Sahakian et al. (1987) | 0.4 mg I/V over 30 mins testing: 15 m + (N=1) | Logical Memory Object Learning | A V | Slight improvement (?sig.) Improvement on one of two testings |
| Stern et al. (1987) | 2–4 mg 0 every 2 hrs. Testing twice daily (N=22) | Selective reminding test Logical Memory Paired-associate learning Visual memory from Wechsler scale | A A A V | No significant effects vs. placebo, though trends for Sis to do best at 3.5 mg/2 hours. |

**Table 7.1 cont.**

| Authors | Dose/Delay till testing | Tests/Ratings | Modality of stimulus | Result |
|---|---|---|---|---|
| Gustafson et al. (1987) | 1.9 mg (approx) I/V infused over 2 hours Testing pre-and during infusion. (N=10) | Paired-associate learning Memory for designs Neuropsychological battery + rCBF measured. | A | No significant effect No significant effect Sig in rCBF in temporal, parietal, occipital regions. |
| Kaye et al. (1982) | THA 30 mg 0 daily (N=10) | Serial learning of word list Selective reminding test | A A | No significant effect No significant effect |
| Summers et al. (1986) | THA 25–200 mg 0 per day after dose titration + lecithin 10.8 g/day (N=15) | Names Learning Orientation test Alzheimer deficit scale | ?A | Significant improvement on all tests, but (?) study not blind (see text) |

*PAL = Paired associate learning.
O = oral adminstration   I/V = intravenous
A = aural                S/C = subcutaneous
V = visual               I/M = intramuscular

improvements are absent, an increase in cerebral blood flow is found (Gustafson *et al.*, 1987). The most promising result has been that obtained in the well-published trial of THA by Summers *et al.*, (1986), in which some quite dramatic benefits were claimed. However, there were a number of technical faults in that trial (Small, Spar and Plotkin, 1987). In particular, it appears that the authors did not actually report the results of the 'blind' phase of their trial, but 'pooled' the findings from a 'blind' and a 'non-blind' phase (Kopelman, 1987).

Following recent reports that 'nicotinic' cholinergic receptors may be depleted in the temporal lobes of Alzheimer patients (Flynn and Mash, 1986; Perry *et al.*, 1987), whilst post-synaptic 'muscarinic' cholinergic receptors are preserved (Mash, Flynn, and Potter, 1985; Perry *et al.*, 1987), there have been two preliminary studies of the effect of nicotine administered to Alzheimer patients. One of these studies reported 'a modest facilitation of memory' (Newhouse *et al.*, 1986), and the other an improvement in tests of attention and information-processing (Jones *et al.*, 1989), consistent with earlier work in healthy subjects (Wesnes and Revell, 1984).

### GABA

Piracetam (1 – acetamide – 2 – pyrrolidine) is a cyclical derivative of GABA, with a chemical structure very similar to GABA. It is believed to increase cerebral energy metabolism (as measured by the turnover of adenosine triphosphate, glucose, and oxygen), and animal studies suggested that it might improve learning (Bartus *et al.*, 1983). However, findings in studies of Alzheimer patients have been disappointing (McDonald, 1982; Branconnier, 1983). On the basis of animal studies, it was also believed that it might potentiate the action of cholinergic agents, when administered together, but a careful study of combined piracetam and lecithin failed to find any significant benefit in Alzheimer patients (Growdon *et al.*, 1986). To the author's knowledge, there have not yet been any trials of piracetam in Huntington patients, in whom GABA is also depleted.

As mentioned above, the effects of benzodiazepines appear to be somewhat paradoxical in that they both facilitate the action of GABA and cause amnesia. Benzodiazepine-induced amnesia has been put forward as a 'model' of the anterograde memory deficit in the Korsakoff syndrome (Brown *et al.*, 1982; Lister and Weingartner, 1987), but, as far as the author is aware, there have not yet been any clinical trials of benzodiazepine-antagonists in either this condition or in the dementias.

### Adrenergic agents

As mentioned above, vasopressin is thought to modulate the action of the noradrenergic neurotransmitters system, but it is controversial whether any cognitive benefits it produces are mediated by an action on attention or memory. There have been several studies of its effect in patients who have dementing or other memory disorders. Several have reported negative results (e.g. Fewtrell *et al.*, 1982) whilst others have obtained an improvement in mood or attention which might account for any benefit in memory (e.g. Oliveros *et al.*, 1978). The most impressive results have been obtained in studies in which either the patients had diabetes insipidus, in which vasopressin is deficient (e.g. Laczi *et al.*, 1982), or a conditioning procedure was employed, i.e. a closer analogue of De Wied's animal studies (e.g. Anderson, David and Bonnel, 1979).

In a series of papers, McEntee and Mair have argued that noradrenergic depletion may be critical to the memory deficit of the alcoholic Korsakoff syndrome (McEntee and Mair, 1978; McEntee *et al.*, 1984), although they qualify this by arguing that this effect is produced by an impairment of attention and arousal (Mair and McEntee, 1983). In two studies, they have reported small but statistically significant benefits in Korsakoff patients at tests of memory and attention, following the administration of a low dose of clonidine (McEntee and Mair 1979; Mair and McEntee, 1986). A puzzle is that they obtained this benefit in Korsakoff patients at the same dose of clonidine at which Frith, Ferrier and Crow (1985) obtained impairment in healthy subjects.

Following Mair and McEntee's work, O'Donnell, Pitts and Fann (1986) compared the effect of *acute* administration of physostigmine or methylphenidate (an adrenergic agent) in six Korsakoff patients, and of *prolonged* administration of choline, methylphenydate, or combined treatment. In the acute phase of the trial, there were no significant drug effects. In the 'chronic' phase, all six patients showed improved performance on a memory test (the 'selective reminding' task) relative to placebo when on methylphenidate, and five out of six patients when on choline. The methylphenidate result was statistically significant (p <0.05), whilst the choline result failed to reach significance. Unfortunately, only one cognitive measure was employed, and the clinical description of the patients was rather sparse.

In Alzheimer patients, Tariot *et al.*, (1987) have recently conducted a trial of L-deprenyl, a monoamine oxidane inhibitor which is metabolized to amphetamine and methamphetamine. They obtained a small but statistically significant improvement in performance at a free recall test, associated with increased energy and social interaction and diminished anxiety in their subjects. The authors suggested that the drug may have enhanced 'effort' or attention.

## CONCLUSIONS

There is now considerable knowledge about the pattern of memory deficits occurring in Korsakoff's syndrome, Alzheimer-type dementia, and Huntington's disease. The use of drugs which modulate different neurotransmitter systems provides a tool for exploring the putative neuropharmacology of these disorders. Anti-cholinergic agents and the benzodiazepine group of drugs both produce a pattern of anterograde amnesia which resembles that seen in the organic amnesic syndrome, but they do not produce any retrograde deficit, nor do they mimic the deficits of working memory and semantic memory seen in dementia. The effects of adrenergic agents have been studied in less detail, but it seems likely that their primary effect is on mechanisms mediating attention and arousal.

The amnesic property of anti-cholinergic agents is consistent with the finding of widespread cholinergic depletion in Alzheimer-type dementia and of possible cholinergic depletion in the alcoholic Korsakoff syndrome. Similarly, the presence of noradrenergic depletion in Alzheimer dementia is consistent with the deficit of attention and arousal which occurs in that condition; and its possible depletion in Korsakoff's syndrome may be related to the characteristic apathy seen in many such patients. More paradoxical is the depletion of GABA which occurs in Alzheimer's and Huntington's dementia, since the benzodiazepines produce amnesia whilst potentiating the action of GABA. This suggests that GABA depletion may not be relevant to the memory disorder of dementia.

Studies of the effect of cholinergic and adrenergic agents administered to amnesic or dementing patients indicate that they can sometimes produce measurable benefits on tests of memory or attention, but these benefits tend to be too small and fickle to be of any great clinical importance. Piracetam, a GABA-like compound, does not appear to produce any benefits, consistent with the view that GABA depletion may not contribute to the memory disorder of dementia.

Administering cholinergic agents directly into the brain's ventricular system does not appear to amplify any benefit from these drugs, which suggests that transplantation of cholinergic or other neuro-hormonal tissue may not be any more successful. There are at least two possible reasons for these disappointing results: (1) Cholinergic depletion may not account for many of the memory deficits seen in dementia, or for the extensive retrograde impairment which occurs in the Korsakoff syndrome (cf. Kopelman and Corn, 1988). (2) Administration of neurotransmitter agents can be of only limited benefit in the presence of neuronal loss, and an effective therapeutic agent will need to suppress the causes of such structural change. Nevertheless, psychopharmacological research of the type described enables us to explore the functional roles of different neurotransmitter substances with much greater precision than in the past; and it may eventually allow a much better understanding of the pathogenesis of psychological deficits and of appropriate avenues for remediation.

## REFERENCES

Albert, M.S., Butters, N. and Brandt, J. (1981) Patterns of remote memory in amnesic and demented patients. *Archives of Neurology,* **38,** 495–500.

Aminoff, M.J., Marshall, J. Smith, E.M. and Wyke, M.A. (1975) Pattern of intellectual impairment in Huntington's Chorea. *Psychological Medicine,* **5,** 169–72.

Anderson, L.T., David, R., Bonnet, K. and Dancis, J. (1979) Passive avoidance learning in Lesch-Nyhan disease: effect of 1 desamino 8 arginine vasopressin. *Life Sciences,* **24,** 905–10.

Arendt, T., Bigl, V., Arendt, A. and Tennstedt, A. (1983) Loss of neurons in the nucleus basalis of Meynert in Alzheimer's disease, paralysis agitans and Korsakoff's disease. *Acta Neuropathologica (Berlin),* **61,** 101–8.

Ashford, J.W. Soldinger, S. Schaffer, J. Cochran, L. Jarvik, L.F. (1981), Physostigmine and its effect on six patients with dementia. *American Journal of Psychiatry,* **138,** 829–30.

Baddeley, A.D. and Warrington, E.K. (1970) Amnesia, and the distinction between long and short-term memory. *Journal of Verbal Learning and Verbal Behaviour,* **9,** 176–89.

Baddeley, A.D. and Wilson, B. (1987) Amnesia, autobiographical memory and confabulation. In D. Rubin (Ed) *Autobiographical Memory.* Cambridge University Press, Cambridge.

Baddeley, A.D., Harris, J.E., Sunderland, A., Watts, K. and Wilson, B. (1987). Closed head injury and memory. In H. Levin (ed.) *Neurobehavioural Recovery from Head Injury.* Oxford University Press, Oxford.

Bartus, R.T., Dean, R.L. and Beer, B. (1983) An evaluation of drugs for improving memory in aged monkeys: implications for clinical trials in humans. *Psychopharmacology Bulletin,* **19,** 168–84.

Bartus, R.T., Dean, R.L., Beer, B. and Lippa, A.S. (1982) The cholinergic hypothesis of geriatric memory dysfunction. *Science,* **217,** 408–17.

Beatty, W.W., Butters, N. and Janowsky, D.S. (1986) Patterns of memory failure after scopolamine treatment: implications for cholinergic hypotheses of dementia, *Behavioural and Neurological Biology,* **45,** 196–11.

Beatty, W.W., Salmon, D.P., Butters, N., Heindel, W.C. and Granholm, E.L. (1988) Retrograde amnesia in patients with Alzheimer's disease or Huntington's disease. *Neurobiology of Ageing,* **9,** 181–6.

Becker, J.T., Boller, F., Saxton, J. and McGonicle-Gibson, K.L. (1987) Normal rates of forgetting of verbal and non-verbal material in Alzheimer's disease. *Cortex,* **23,** 59–72.

Beller, S.A., Overall, J.E. and Swann, A.C. (1985). Efficacy of oral physostigmine in primary degenerative dementia. *Psychopharmacology,* **87,** 147–51.

Blackwood, D.H.R. and Christie, J.E (1986). The effects of physostigmine and auditory P300 in Alzheimer-type dementia. *Biological Psychiatry*, **21**, 557–60.

Boyd, W., Graham-White, J., Blackwood, G., Glen, I. and McQueen, J. (1977) Clinical effects of choline in Alzheimer senile dementia. *Lancet*, **2**, 711.

Branconnier, R.J. (1983) The efficacy of the cerebral metabolic enhancers in the treatment of senile dementia. *Psychopharmacology Bulletin*, **19**, 212–19.

Brooks, D.N. and Baddeley, A.D. (1976) What can amnesic patients learn? *Neuropsychologia*, **14**, 111–22.

Brown, J. (1958), Some tests of the decay theory of immediate memory. *Quarterly Journal of Experimental Psychology*, **10**, 12–21.

Brown, J., Lewis, V., Brown, M., Horn, G. and Bowes, J.B. (1982) A comparison between transient amnesias induced by two drugs (Diazepam or Lorazepam) and amnesia of organic origin. *Neuropsychologia*, **20**, 55–70.

Brown, J., Brown, M.W. and Bowes, J.B. (1983) Effects of Lorazepam on rate of forgetting, on retrieval from semantic memory and on manual dexterity. *Neuropsychologia*, **21**, 501–12.

Bruno, G., Mohr, E., Gillespie, M., Fedio, P. and Chase, T.N., (1986) Muscarinic agonist therapy of Alzheimer's disease: a clinical trial of RS-86 *Archives of Neurology*, **43** 659–61.

Butters, N. and Cermak, L.S. (1980) *Alcoholic Korsakoff's Syndrome: an information-processing approach to amnesia*. Academic Press; New York.

Butters, N., Granholm, E., Salmon, D., Grant, I. and Wolfe, J. (1987) Episodic and semantic memory – a comparison of amnesic and demented patients. *Journal of Clinical and Experimental Neuropsychology*, **9**, 479–97.

Caine, E.D., Weingartner, H., Ludlow, C.L., Cudahy, E.A. and Wehry, S. (1981) Qualitative analysis of scopolamine-induced amnesia. *Psychopharmacology*, **74**, 74–80.

Christie, J.E., Shering, A., Ferguson, G. and Glen, A.I.M. (1981) Physostigmine and arecoline: effects of intravenous infusions in Alzheimer pre-senile dementia. *British Journal of Psychiatry*, **138**, 46–50.

Clark, A.W., Parhad, I.M., Folstein, S.E., Whitehouse, P.J., Herdeen, J.C., Price, D.L. and Chase, G.A. (1983) The nucleus basalis in Huntington's disease. *Neurology*, **33** 1262–7.

Clark, C.R., Geffen, G.M. and Geffen L.B. (1986) Role of monoamine pathways in attention and effort. *Psychopharmacology*, **90**, 35–9.

Corkin, S. (1982) Some relationships between global amnesias and the memory impairments in Alzheimer's disease. In: S. Corkin, K.L. Davis, J.H. Growdon, E. Usdin and R.J. Wurtman (Eds) *Alzheimer's disease: a report of research in progress*. Raven Press; New York.

Crow, T.J. and Grove-White, I.G. (1973) An analysis of the learning deficit following hyoscine administration to man. *British Journal of Pharmacology*, **49**, 322–7.

208    *The psychopharmacology of memory disorders*

Crow, T.J., Grove-White, I.G. and Ross, D.G. (1975) The specificity of the action of hyoscine on human learning. *British Journal of Clinical Pharmacology*, **2**, 367–8.

Curran, H.V. (1986) Tranquilising memories: a review of the effects of benzodiazepines on human memory. *Biological Psychology*, **23**, 179–213.

Curran, H.V., Schiwy, W. and Lader, M., (1987) Differential amnesic properties. *Psychopharmacology*, **92**, 358–64.

Dannebaum, S.E., Parkinson, S.R. and Inman, V.W. (1988) Short-term forgetting: comparisons between patients with dementia of the Alzheimer type, depressed, and normal elderly. *Cognitive Neuropsychology*, **5**, 213–33.

Davis, K.L., Mohs, R.C. (1982) Enhancement of memory processes in Alzheimer's disease with multiple-dose intravenous physostigmine. *American Journal of Psychiatry*, **139**, 1421–4.

Davis, K.L., Mohs, R.C, Rosen, W.G., Greenwald, B.S., Levy, M.I. and Horvarth, T.B, (1983) Memory enhancement with oral physostigmine in Alzheimer's desease. *New England Journal of Medicine*, **308**, 721.

De Wied, D. (1984) The importance of vasopressin in memory. *Trends in Neuroscience*, **7**, 62–4.

De Wied, D. and Van Ree, J.M. (1982) Neuropeptides, mental performance, and ageing. *Life Sciences*, **31**, 709–19.

Dorow, R, Berenberg, D, Duka, T. and Sauerbrey, N. (1987) Amnestic effects of lormetazepam and their reversal by the benzodiazepine antagonist RO15–17 88. *Psychopharmacology*, **93**, 507–14.

Drachman, D. and Arbitt, J. (1966) Memory and the hippocampal complex. *Archives of Neurology*, **15**, 52–61.

Drachman, D.A. and Leavitt, J. (1974) Human memory and the cholinergic system. *Archives of Neurology*, **30**, 113–21.

Drachman, D.A., Noffsinger, D., Sahakian, B.J., Kurdziel, S. and Fleming, P. (1980) Ageing, memory, and the cholinergic system. *Neurobiology of Ageing*, **1**, 39–43.

Dubois, B., Danze, F., Pillon, B., Cusimano, G., Lhermitte, F. and Agid, Y. (1987) Cholinergic-dependent cognitive deficits in Parkinson's disease. *Annals of Neurology*, **22**, 26–30.

Dunne, M.P. and Hartley, L.R. (1985) The effects of scopolamine upon verbal memory: evidence for an attentional hypothesis. *Acta Psychologica*, **58**, 205–17.

Dunne, M.P. and Hartley, L.R. (1986) Scopolamine and the control of attention in humans. *Psychopharmacology*, **89**, 94–7.

Eslinger, P.J. and Damasio, A.R. (1986) Preserved motor learning in Alzheimer's disease: implications for anatomy and behaviour. *Journal of Neuroscience*, **6**, 3006–9.

Etienne, P., Cauthier, S., Johnson, G., Collier, B., Mendis, T., Dastorr, D., Cole, M. and Muller, H. (1978) Clinical effects of acetylcholine in Alzheimer's disease. *Lancet*, **1**, 508–9.

Fewtrell, W.D., House, A.O., Jamie, P.F., Oates, M.R. and Cooper, J.E., (1982) Effects of vasopressin on memory and new learning in a brain-injured population. *Psychological Medicine,* **12** 423–25.

Flynn, D.D. and Mash, D.C. (1986) Characterisation of L – [3H] nicotine binding in human cerebral cortex: comparison between Alzheimer's disease and the normal. *Journal of Neurochemistry,* **47,** 1948–54.

Frith, C.D., Richardson, J.T.E., Samuel, M., Crow, T.J. and McKenna, P.J. (1984) The effects of intravenous diazepam and hyoscine upon human memory. *Quarterly Journal of Experimental Psychology,* **36A,** 133–44.

Frith, C.D., J. Ferrier, I.N. and Crow, T.J. (1985) Selective impairment of paired associate learning after administration of a centrally-acting adrenergic agonist (clonidine) *Psychopharmacology,* **87,** 490–93.

Gash, D.M. and Thomas, G.J. (1983) What is the importance of vasopressin in memory processes? *Trends in Neurosciences,* **6,** 197–8.

Ghoneim, M.M. and Mewaldt, S.P. (1975) Effects of diazepam and scopolamine on storage, retrieval, and organisational processes in memory. *Psychopharmacologia (Berlin),* **44,** 257–62.

Ghoneim, M.M. and Mewaldt, S.P. (1977) Studies on human memory: the interaction of diazepam, scopolamine, and physostigmine. *Psychopharmacology,* **52,** 1–6.

Ghoneim, M.M., Mewaldt, S.P. and Henrichs, J.R. (1984) Dose-response analysis of the behavioural effects of diazepam: 1 learning and memory. *Psychopharmacology,* **82,** 291–5.

Graf, P., Squire, L.R. and Mandler, G. (1984) The information that amnesic patients do not forget. *Journal of Experimental Psychology: Language, Memory and Cognition,* **10,** 164–78.

Grober, E., (1985) Encoding of item-specific information in Alzheimer's disease. *Journal of Clinical and Experimental Neuropsychology,* **7,** 614.

Growdon, J.H., Corkin, S., Huff, F.J. and Rosen, T.J. (1986) Piracetam with lecithin in the treatment of Alzheimer's disease. *Neurobiology of Ageing,* **7,** 269–76.

Gustafson, L., Edvinsson, L., Dahlgren, N., Hagberg, B., Risberg, J., Rosen, I. and Ferno, H. (1987) Intravenous physostigmine treatment of Alzheimer's disease evaluated by psychometric testing, regional cerebral blood flow (rCBF) measurement, and EEG. *Psychopharmacology,* **93,** 31–5.

Hart, S., Smith, C.M. and Swash, M. (1988) Word fluency in patients with early dementia of Alzheimer type. *British Journal of Clinical Psychology,* **27,** 115–24.

Heyman, A., Schmechel, D., Wilkinson, W., Roger, H., Krishnan, R., Holloway, D., Schultz, K., Gwyther, L, Peoples, R., Utley, C., and others (1987) Failure of long-term high-dose lecithin to retard the progression of early-onset Alzheimer's disease. *Journal of Neurotransmission (Supplement),* **24,** 279–86.

Hollander, E., Davidson, M., Mohs, R.C., Hovarth, T.B., Davis, B.M., Zemishlany, Z. and Davis, K.L. (1987) RS-86 in the treatment of Alzheimer's disease: cognitive and biological effects. *Biological Psychiatry,* **22,** 1067–78.

Hollander, E., Mohs, R.C., Davis, K.L. (1986) Cholinergic approaches to the treatment of Alzheimer's disease. *British Medical Bulletin*, **42**, 97–100.

Huff, F.J., Corkin, S. and Growdon, J.H. (1986) Semantic impairment and anomia in Alzheimer's disease. *Brain and Language*, **28**, 235–49.

Huppert, F.A. (1991) Age-related changes in memory: learning and remembering new information. In F. Boller and J. Grafman (eds) *Handbook of Neuropsychology*, Elsevier, **5**, (7) 123–47.

Huppert, F.A. and Piercy, M. (1978) Dissociation between learning and remembering in organic amnesia. *Nature*, **275**, 317–18.

Johns, C.A., Greenwald, B.S., Mohs, R.C. and Davis, K.L. (1983) The cholinergic treatment strategy in ageing and senile dementia. *Psychopharmacology Bulletin*, **19**, 185–97.

Jones, G., Sahakian, B.J. Levy, R., Gray, J. and Warburton, D.W. (1989) The effects of nicotine on attention, information processing, and short-term memory in patients with dementia of the Alzheimer type. *British Journal of Psychiatry*, **54**, 797–800.

Jotkowitz, S., (1983) Lack of clinical efficacy of chronic oral physostigmine in Alzheimer's disease. *Annals of Neurology*, **14**, 690–1.

Kasniak, A., Garron, D. and Fox, J. (1979) Differential effects of age and cerebral atrophy upon span of immediate recall and paired-associate learning in older patients suspected of dementia. *Cortex*, **15**, 285–95.

Kaye, W.H., Sitaram, N., Weingartner, H., Ebert, M.H., Smallsberg, S. and Gillin, J.C. (1982) Modest facilitation of memory in dementia with combined lecithin and anticholinesterase treatment. *Biological Psychiatry*, **51**, 275–9.

Knopman, D.S. and Nissen, M.J. (1987) Implicit learning in patients with probable Alzheimer's disease. *Neurology*, **37**, 784–8.

Kopelman, M.D. (1985) Rates of forgetting in Alzheimer-type dementia and Korsakoff's syndrome. *Neuropsychologia*, **23**, 623–38.

Kopelman, M.D. (1986a) Recall of anomalous sentences in dementia and amnesia. *Brain and Language*, **29**, 154–70.

Kopelman, M.D. (1986b) The cholinergic neurotransmitter system in human memory and dementia: a review, *Quarterly Journal of Experimental Psychology*, **38A**, 535–73.

Kopelman, M.D. (1987) Oral tetrahydroaminoacridine in the treatment of senile dementia, Alzheimer's type (correspondence). *New England Journal of Medicine*, **316**, 1604.

Kopelman, M.D. (1989) Remote and autobiographical memory, temporal context memory, and frontal atrophy in Korsakoff and Alzheimer patients. *Neuropsychologia*, **27**, 437–60.

Kopelman, M.D. and Lishman, W.A. (1986) Pharmacological treatment of dementia (non-cholinergic). *British Medical Bulletin*, **42**, 101–5.

Kopelman, M.D. and Corn, T.H. (1988) Cholinergic 'blockade' as a model comparison of the memory deficits with those of Alzheimer-type dementia and the alcoholic Korsakoff syndrome. *Brain*, **111**, 1079–110.

Kopelman, M.D., Wilson, B. and Baddeley, A.D. (1989) The autobiographical memory interview: a new assessment of autobiographical and personal semantic memory in amnesic patients. *Journal of Clinical Experimental Neuropsychology*, **11**, 724–44.

Laczi, F., Valkusz, Z., Laszlo, F.A., Wagner, A., Jardanhazy, T., Szasz, A., Szilard, J., Teledgdy, G., (1982) Effects of lysine-vasopressin and 1 deamino 8D arginine vasopressin on men in healthy individuals and diabetes insipidus patients *Psychoneuroendocrinology*, **7**, 185–93.

Lister, R.G. and Weingartner, H.J. (1987) Neuropharmacological strategies for understanding psychobiologcial determinants of cognition. *Human-Neurobiology*, **6**, 119–27.

Little, A., Levy, R., Chuaqui-Kidd, P. and Hand, D. (1985) A double blind placebo controlled trial of high dose lecithin in Alzheimer's disease. *Journal of Neurology, Neurosurgery and Psychiatry*, **48**, 736–42.

Mair, R.G. and McEntee, W.J. (1983) Korsakoff's psychosis noradrenergic systems and cognitive impairment. *Behavioural Brain Research*, **9**, 1–32.

Mair, R.G. and McEntee, W.J. (1986) Cognitive enhancement in Korsakoff's psychosis by clonidine; a comparison with L-dopa and ephedrine. *Psychopharmacology*, **88**, 374–80.

Martin, A., Brouwers, P., Cox, C. and Fedio, P. (1985) On the nature of the verbal memory deficit in Alzheimer's disease. *Brain and Languages*, **25**, 323–41.

Martone, M., Butters, N., Payne, M., Becker, J.T. and Sax, D.S. (1984) Dissociations between skill learning and verbal recognition amnesia and dementia, *Archives of Neurology*, **41**, 965–70.

Martone, M., Butters, N. and Trauner, D. (1986) Some analyses of forgetting of pictorial material in amnesic and demented patients, *Journal of Clinical and Experimental Neuropsyshology*, **8**, 161–78.

Mash, D.C., Flynn, D.D. and Potter, L.T. (1985) Loss of M2 muscarinic receptors in the cerebral cortex in Alzheimer's disease and exceptional cholinergic denervation. *Science*, **228**, 1115–17.

McDonald, R.J (1982) Drug treatment of senile dementia. In: D Wheatley (Ed.,) *Psychopharmacology of Old Age*. Oxford University Press, pp. 113–37.

Mc Entee, W.J. and Mair, R.G (1978) Memory impairment in Korsakoff's psychosis a correlation with brain noradrenergic activity. *Science*, **202**, 905–7.

McEntee, W.J. and Mair, R.G. (1979) Memory enhancement in Korsakoff's psychosis by clonidine: further evidence for a noradrenergic deficit. *Annals of Neurology*, **7**, 466–70.

McEntee, W.J., Mair, R.G and Langlais. P.J. (1984) Neurochemical pathology in Korsakoff's psychosis: implications for others cognitive disorders, *Neurology*, **34**, 648–52.

Meudell, P.R., Butters, N. and Montgomery, K. (1978) The role rehearsal in the short-term memory performance of patients with Korsakoff's and Huntington's disease. *Neuropsychologia*, **16**, 507–10.

Miller, E., (1975) Impaired recall and the memory disturbance in presenile dementia. *British Journal of Social and Clinical Psychology*, **14** 73–79.

Millar, K., Jeffcoate, W.J. and Walden, C.P. (1987) Vasporessin and memory improvement in normal short-term recall and reduction of alcohol-induced amnesia, *Psychology Medicine*, **17**, 335–41.

Mohs, R.C., Davis, B.M., John, C.A., Mathe, A.A., Greenwald, B.S., Horvarth, T.B. and Davis, K.L. (1985) Oral physostigmine treatment of patients with Alzheimers's disease. *American Journal of Psychiatry*, **142**, 28–33.

Morris, R.G. (1984) Dementia and the functioning of the articulatory loop system, *Cognitive Neuropsychology*, **1**, 143–57.

Morris, R.G. (1986) Short-term forgetting in senile dementia of the Alzheimer's type. *Cognitive Neuropsychology*, **3**, 77–97.

Morris, R.G., Wheatley, J. and Britton, P.G. (1983) Retrieval from long-term memory in senile dementia: cued recall revisited. *British Journal of Clinical Psychology* **22**, 141–2.

Morris, R.G and Kopelman, M.D. (1986) The memory deficits in Alzheimer-type dementia: a review. *Quarterly Journal of Experimental Psychology*, **38A**, 575–602

Muramato, O., Sugishita., M., and Ando, K., (1984) Cholinergic system and constructional praxis: a further study of physostigmine in Alzheimer's disease. *Journal of Neurology, Neurosurgery, and Psychiatry*, **47**, 485–91.

Muramato, O., Sugishitam, M., Sugita, H. and Toyokura, Y. (1979) Effect of physostigmine on constructional and memory tasks in Alzheimer's disease. *Archives of Neurology* **36**, 501–3.

Nebes, R.D., Martin, D.C., Horn, L.C. (1984) Sparing of semantic memory in Alzheimer's disease. *Journal of Abnormal Psychology*, **9**, 321–30.

Newhouse, P.A. Sunderland, T., Thompson, K., Tariot, P.N., Weingartner, H., Mueller, E.R., Cohen, R.M. and Murphy D.L. (1986) Intravenous nicotine in a patient with Alzheimer's disease (letter) *American Journal of Psychiatry*, **143** 1494–9.

Nissen, M.J., Knopman, D.S and Schacter, D.L. (1987) Neurochemical dissociation of memory systems. *Neurology*, **37**, 789–94.

Nuotto, E. (1983) Psychomotor, physiological and cognitive effects of scopolamine and ephedrine in healthy man. *European Journal of Clinical Pharmacology*, **24**, 603–9.

Ober, B.A., Dronkers, N.F., Koss, E., Delis, D.C and Friedland, R.P. (1986) Retrieval from semantic memory in Alzheimer-type dementia. *Journal of Clinical and Experimental Neuropsychology*, **8**, 75–92.

O'Boyle, C., Barry, H., Fox, E., Harris, D., McCreary, C. (1987) Benzodiazepine-induced event amnesia following a stressful surgical procedure. *Psychopharmacology*, **91**, 244–7.

O.Donnell, V.M., Pitts, W.M. and Fann, W.E. (1986) Noradrenergic and cholinergic agents in Korsakoff's syndrome. *Clinical Neuropharmacology*, **9**, 65–70.

Oliveros, J.C., Jandali, M.K., Timset-Berthier, M., Remy, R., Benghezal, A.M, Audibert, A. and Moeglen, J.M. (1978) Vasopressin in amnesia. *Lancet*, **i**, 42.

Parrott, A.C. (1986) The effects of transdermal scopolamine and 4 dose levels of oral scopolamine (0.15, 0.3, 0.6 and 1.2 mg) upon psychological performance. *Psychopharmacology*, 89, 347–54.

Penn, R.D., Martin, E.M., Wilson, R.S., Fox, J.H and Savoy, S.M. (1988) Intraventricular bethanechol infusion for Alzheimer's disease: results of double-blind and escalating-dose trials. *Neurology*, **38**, 219–22.

Perry, T.L. Hansten, S. and Kloster, M., (1973) Huntington's chorea: deficiency of gamma-amino-butyric acid in brain. *New England Journal of Medicine*, **288**, 337–42.

Perry, E.K, Perry, R.H., Smith, C.J., Dick, D.J., Candy, J.M., Edwardson, J.H., Fairburn, A. and Blessed, G., (1987) Nicotinic receptor abnormalities in Alzheimer's and Parkinson's disease. *Journal of Neurology, Neurosurgery, and Psychiatry*, **50**, 806–9.

Peters, B.H. and Levin, H.S. (1977) Memory enhancement after physostigmine treatment in the amnesic syndrome, *Archives of Neurology* **34**, 215–19.

Peters, B.H. and Levin, H.S., (1979) Effects of physostigmine and lecithin on memory in Alzheimer's disease. *Annals of Neurology*, **6**, 219–21.

Peterson, L.R. and Peterson. M. J., (1959) Short-term retention for individual items. *Journal of Experimental Psychology*, **58**, 193–8.

Rossor, M.N. Garrett, N.J., Johnson, A. L., Mountjoy, C.Q., Roth, M. and Iverson L.L. (1982) A post-mortem study of the cholinergic and Gaba systems in senile dementia. *Brain*, **105**, 313–30.

Rossor, M. and Iversen, L.L., (1986) Non-cholinergic neurotransmitter abnormalities in Alzheimer's disease. *British Medical Bulletin*, **42**, 70–4.

Rossor, M.N., Iversen, L.L., Reynolds, G.P., Mountjoy, C.Q. and Roth, M. (1984) Neurochemical characteristics of early and late onset types of Alzheimer's disease. *British Medical Journal*, **288**, 961–4.

Russell, W.R. and Smith.A. (1961) Post-traumatic amnesia in closed head injury. *Archives of Neurology*, **5**, 4–29.

Safer, D.M. and Allen, R.P. (1971) The central effects of scopolamine in man. *Biological Psychiatry*, **3**, 347–55.

Sagar, H.J., Cohen, N.J., Sullivan, E.V., Corkin, S. and Growdon, J.H. (1988) Remote memory function in Alzheimer's disease and Parkinson's disease. *Brain*, **111**, 185–206.

Sahakian, B. J., Joyce, E. M. and Lishman, W.A., (1987). Cholinergic effects on constructional abilities and mnemonic processes: a case report. *Psychological Medicine*, **17**, 329–33.

Sahgal, A. (1984) A critique of the vasopressin-memory hypothesis, *Psychopharmacology*, **83**, 215–28.

Shimamura, A.P. and Squire, L.R. (1986) Korsakoff's syndrome: a study of the relation between anterograde amnesia and remote memory impairment. *Behavioral Neuroscience*, **100**, 165–70.

214     *The psychopharmacology of memory disorders*

Shimamura, A.P., Salmon, D.P. and Squire, L.R. (1987) Memory dysfunctions and word priming in dementia and amnesia. *Behavioural
Neuroscience*, **101**, 347–51.
Signoret, J.L., Whiteley, A. and Lhermitte, F. (1978) Influence of choline
on amnesia in early Alzheimer's disease. *Lancet*, **2**, 837.
Small, G.W., Spar, J.E. and Plotkin, D.A. (1987) Oral tetrahydroaminoacridine in the treatment of senile dementia, Alzheimer's type.
(correspondence). *New England Journal of Medicine*, **316**, 1604.
Smith, C. M. and Swash, M, (1979) Physostigmine in Alzheimer's
disease. *Lancet*, **1**, 42.
Smith, C.M., Swash, M., Exton-Smith, A., Phillips, M., Overstall, P.,
Piper, M. and Bailey, M. (1978) Choline therapy in Alzheimer's
disease, *Lancet*, **2**, 318
Snel, J., Taylor, J. and Wegman, M., (1987) Does DGAVP influ-
ence memory, attention and mood in young healthy men.
*Psychopharmacology*, **92**, 224–8.
Spinnler, H., Della Sala, S., Bandera, S. and Baddeley, A.D. (1988)
Dementia, ageing, and the structure of human memory. *Cognitive
Neuropsychology*, **5**, 193–211.
Stern, Y., Sano, M. and Mayeux, R., (1987) Effects of oral physostigmine
in Alzheimer's disease. *Annals of Neurology*, **22**, 306–10.
Sullivan, E.V., Shedlack, K.J., Corkin, S. and Growdon, J.H. (1982)
Physostigmine and lecithin in Alzheimer's disease. In *Alzheimer's
Disease: a report on progress in research*, S. Corkin, J.H. Growdon, E.
Usdin and R.J. Wurtman (eds) *Ageing* **14**. Raven Press, New York.
Sullivan, E.V., Corkin, S. and Growdon, J.H. (1986) Verbal and non-
verbal short-term memory in patients with Alzheimer's disease
and in healthy elderly subjects. *Developmental Neuropsychology*, **2**,
387–400.
Summers, W.K., Majovski, L.V., Marsh, G.M. Tachiki, K. and Kling,
A. (1986) Oral tetrahydroaminoacridine in long-term treatment of
senile dementia Alzheimer type. *New England Journal of Medicine*,
**315**, 1241–5.
Sunderland, T., Tariot, P.N., Cohen, R.M. Weingartner, H., Mueller,
E.A. and Murphy, D.L. (1987) Anticholinergic sensitivity in patients
with dementia of the Alzheimer-type and age-matched controls: a
dose-response curve. *Archives of General Psychiatry*, **44**, 418–25.
Tariot, P.N., Sunderland, T., Weingartner, H., Murphy, D.L., Welko-
witz, J.A., Thompson, K. and Cohen, R.M. (1987) Cognitive
effects of L-deprenyl in Alzheimer's disease. *Psychopharmacology*,
**91**, 489–95.
Thal, L.J., Fuld, P.A, Masur, D.M., and Sharpless, N.S. (1983) Oral physostigmine and lecithin improve memory in Alzheimer's disease.
*Annals of Neurology*, **13**, 491–6.
Thomlinson, B.E., and Corsellis, J.A.N. (1984) Ageing and the
dementias. In J.H. Adams, J.A.N. Corsellis and L. W. Duchen (Eds)
*Greenfield's Neuropathology*, 4th ed. Edward Arnold, London.
Warrington, E.K. and Weiskrantz, L. (1970) Amnesic syndrome:
consolidation or retrieval? *Nature*, **228**, 628–30.

Weiner, N. (1980) Atropine, scopolamine, and related antimuscarinic drugs. In A.G. Gilman, L.S. Goodman and A. Gilman (Eds) *Goodman and Gilman's The Pharmacological Basis of Therapeutics*, Sixth Edition. Macmillan: New York. Balliere Tindall: London, pp. 120–37.

Weingartner, H., Golp. P., Ballenger, J.C., Smallberg, S.A., Summers, R., Rubinow, D.R., Post, R.M. and Goodwin, F.K. (1981) Effects of vasopressin on human memory functions: *Science*, **211**, 601–3.

Wesnes K. and Revell P. (1984) The separate and combined effects of scopolamine and nicotine on human information processing. *Psychopharmacology*, **84**, 5–11

Wesnes, K. and Warburton, D.M. (1983) Effects of scopolamine on stimulus sensitivity and response bias in a visual vigilance task, *Neuropsychobiology*, **9**, 154–7.

Wesnes, K. and Warburton, D.M. (1984) Effects of scopolamine and nicotine on human rapid information processing performance. *Psychopharmacology*, **82**, 147–50.

Wesnes, K., Simpson, P. and Kidd, A. (1988) An investigation of the range of cognitive impairments induced by scopolamine 0.6mg sc. *Human Psychopharmocology*, **82**, 27–41.

Whitehouse, P.J. (1988) Intraventricular bethanechol in Alzheimer's disease: a continuing controversy. *Neurology*, **38**, 307–8.

Whitehouse, J.R. (1981) Pharmacotherapy for age-related behavioural deficiencies. *Journal of Nervous and Mental Disease*, **169**, 139–55.

Wilson, R.S., Bacon, L.D., Fox, J.H. and Kasdzniak, A.W. (1983) Primary and secondary memory of the Alzheimer-type. *Journal of Clinical Neuropsychology*, **5**, 193–211.

Witt, E.D. (1985) Neuroanatomical consequences of thiamine deficiency: a comparative analysis. *Alcohol 7 Alcoholism* **20**, 201–21.

Zangwill, O.L. (1946) Some qualitative observations on verbal memory in cases of cerebral lesion. *British Journal of Psychology*, **37**, 8–19.

## Chapter 8

# Disorders of attention: their effect on behaviour, cognition and rehabilitation

RODGER Ll. WOOD

### INTRODUCTION

The attentional system is a major control process mediating a number of cognitive functions that underlie many aspects of behaviour. Disorders of attention can be regarded as a fundamental cause of many forms of cognitive impairment and often form the basis of other psychological disorders which follow brain injury. The role of attention in disorders of memory and learning has been recognized for some time, but it has only recently been introduced as a concept important to rehabilitation and the establishment of functional skills. The apparent delay between translating research findings from academic psychology into techniques that can be used in a clinical environment probably owes something to the ambiguity that has always been associated with the attentional process. Psychologists have never provided a clear definition of attention and, to a large extent, this has led to problems identifying or measuring attention (using conventional psychological tests) in a way which distinguishes attentional abnormalities from other forms of cognitive impairment (Lezak, 1983).

The association between brain injury and disorders of attention has been recognized since the beginning of this century (e.g., Meyer, 1904). Early observations of attentional impairment were made in the context of psychological testing when patients showed deficits in mental speed and an inability to sustain attention. More recently, attentional deficits have been observed in a rather broader context. Clinical neuropsychologists regularly encounter head-injured patients who complain of a loss of concentration in a variety of real-life situations, causing disruption at work and in other important activities. Caveness (1969) reported that 41% of soldiers who received head injuries during the Korean war continued to complain of a general difficulty concentrating, five years post injury. Mateer, Sohlberg and Crinean (1987) found that many head injured patients who describe various types of 'forgetting experiences' were actually describing problems of attention and concentration. It was found that the memory problems most frequently experienced related to activities with significant attentional demands.

Hecaen and Albert (1978) comment that disorders of attention are most noticeable in patients who have sustained injury to the frontal regions of the brain, an opinion shared by Stuss and Benson (1986). They describe how the 'attentional circuit' connects with important frontal structures to mediate the integrative and organizational processes and also link with limbic structures and other cortical areas to regulate the flow of information throughout the brain. Stuss and Benson consider that the inflexible, disorganized, fragmented, and concrete style of behaviour that is often seen in association with frontal injury to the brain, results from damage to the fronto-thalamic gating system which controls the ascending reticular activating system (ARAS) and descending fibres from the frontal cortex.

It is clear that a complex feedback network comprises the circuitry for the information processing system of the brain. Damage to this network can lead to a reduction in awareness of, and response to, environmental events that normally act as 'cues' for behaviour. Unfortunately, the information processing system is very vulnerable to the acceleration-deceleration forces and other movement effects that are associated with concussional brain injury (normally seen in the context of road traffic accidents). Teasdale and Mendelow (1984) consider that these concussional forces disrupt the neuronal connections between the frontal cortex and other cerebral mechanisms.

Eames and Wood (1984) argued that disturbances of attention prevent information being processed into 'conscious awareness'. This in turn, interferes with reliable storage of information, probably due to a failure of the mechanisms involved in 'working memory' (Baddeley and Hitch, 1974). This is a stage of memory where information is processed in terms of its meaningfulness for on-going behaviour. Working memory incorporates the concept of a **central executive**. This facilitates temporary storage of information but only within the capacity of the information processing system's ability to divide attention during information processing. The central executive acts as a controller of memory. It allows information to be held in short-term storage while attention is temporarily shifted to other stimuli or ideas. As such, the central executive allows parallel processing of information as well as different levels of processing. Working memory is therefore intrinsic to routine cognitive tasks such as sentence construction, comprehension and problem solving, as well as the speed and accuracy of the way information is processed and acted upon.

Attention can therefore be considered as a thread which runs through the fabric of human life, integrating cognitive and emotional components of social behaviour. It is also a process which is fundamental to new learning, as Wood (1987) showed using a simple discrimination learning task. Therapists and clinicians who are engaged in cognitive rehabilitation need, therefore, to develop an appreciation of the role of attention in order to recognize how it mediates various forms of complex behaviour. This will allow treatment techniques in rehabilitation to be designed and adapted, in order to accommodate individuals with disorders of attention, thereby improving their ability to learn.

### ATTENTION AND LEARNING ABILITY

Rehabilitation relies upon learning for its success. In cases of brain-injury rehabilitation, the learning apparatus (the brain) has been damaged, therefore, the learning process is almost certainly 'disabled'. One theme of this chapter will be to argue that the process of learning relies upon an attentional mechanism which, as stated, is rather vulnerable to the forces which operate in acceleration-deceleration, closed-head concussional injuries. This has been confirmed by a number of clinical and research studies; e.g. Meyer, 1904; Conkey, 1938; Goldstein, 1939; Ruesch, 1944; Denker and Lovfring, 1958; Wood, 1987. More recently such notable specialists as Geschwind (1982) have described attention disorders as one of the most common deficits of higher mental function seen in neurological practice. Newcombe (1985) has also used the concept of attention to describe why brain injured patients appear distractible, fail to respond to environmental cues and show a variability of behaviour, including emotional lability. Mahoney (1974), and Schneider, Dumais and Shiffrin, (1984) also consider attention to exert an important influence upon human behaviour, especially the acquisition and final performance of a new skill.

The main premise underlying this form of reasoning is that attention is generally regarded as a 'control process' mediating many aspects of human behaviour. During the 1930s, behaviour was considered to be a product of stimulus-response contingencies. Any cognitive or 'mentalistic' explanation for behaviour was ignored because it was not directly observable or measurable. Ironically, it was the behaviourists themselves who were forced to re-introduce the concept of attention to try and explain conditioning phenomena that could not be predicted, or directly measured, on the basis of response contiguities.

This chink in the armour of radical behaviourism opened up an opportunity for many aspects of learning to be explained on the basis of cognitive mediators. The role of attention in learning has occupied a fairly central position as one of the main cognitive processes mediating many aspects of human learning (Baron, Myerson and Hale 1988). Wood (1988a) has described the way disorders of attention act as a 'clinical constraint', not only in formal conditioning paradigms (discrimination learning) but also at times when it is necessary to change social behaviour or help a brain-injured patient acquire a functional skill.

ATTENTION AND MEMORY

Atkinson and Shiffrin (1968), and Underwood (1978) considered attention to be the major **control process** in the passage of information into, and out of, memory. This line of thinking emphasizes an important distinction, one which discriminates between the concept of memory as a **system**, and the concept of memory as a series of **structures** or **stores**. The 'memory system' is far more analogous to the concept of attention as a system of information processing. The early information processing models of memory stressed the existence of a series of distinct storage systems through which incoming information flowed. Further research (e.g. Atkinson and Shiffrin, 1968) while accepting the notion of multiple storage, stressed the degree to which the individual can exercise various processing **strategies** which control this flow of information. The degree to which an item of information is remembered is therefore determined not just by the attentional (or structural) capacity of the storage system, but also by the particular control strategies employed by an individual.

Traditionally, there has been a tendency for many individuals to compartmentalize memory into two distinct neuropsychological conditions. This is represented on the one hand by the process of **encoding**, (registering information for future use), while on the other hand 'remembering' is regarded as a process of **retrieval**. However, the evolution of research into human memory has helped many authorities recognize that these two processes are not distinct and separate, but form different stages on a continuum of information processing. Encoding, or the laying down of information for future recall, must take place continuously throughout our everyday lives. This aspect of the memory process should be regarded as an active and variable system, integrated with a number of cognitive activities which underlie and represent human behaviour. Certain forms of information (memory) processing take place at a very conscious level, such as when learning takes place in a formal context (the classroom). In such a setting we make a positive effort to encode information and 'controlled-processing' (Shiffrin and Schneider, 1977) plays an important role (Wood, 1984; 1987).

Not all learning and memorizing occurs in this way however. Most behavioural psychologists would agree that a large part of encoding and retrieval of information occurs involuntarily. During conversation, for example, we seem to become suddenly aware of certain memories which can be used to develop our thinking and add substance to the discussion. Some form of 'search process' must therefore be continuously involved in the operation of retrieval, 'drawing out from memory, information related to the ongoing stream of cognitive activity' (Morris, 1978, p. 64). The thrust of research in cognitive psychology has been centred around the questions 'what directs the search?' and 'what determines the relevance of the retrieved information?' This complex problem has not yet been properly resolved but the arguments cannot be entirely ignored by rehabilitation therapists or neuropsychologists engaged in the amelioration of memory deficits (and related cognitive skills) with survivors of severe brain injury.

To some extent, the arguments revolve around how information is processed. Craik and Lockhart (1972) proposed an argument which suggested that a stimulus was processed through a fixed series of levels (or analysers) from structural to semantic (the depth of processing arguments). Later work however, such as that by Craik and Tulving (1975), and Lockhart, Craik and Jacoby (1976) have expressed dissatisfaction with a simple depth of processing analogy, because it is difficult to conceptualize a continuum of cognitive analysis which allows a shading of structural analysis into semantic analysis.

The more recent proposals are of **domains** of encoding, with a separate system of processing in each domain. No single domain relies on a full structural analysis of the information before semantic processing can begin. This introduces a process whereby the familiarity of a stimulus (e.g. a familiar phrase, person, or object) is related to the extent or complexity of its processing requirements. Familiar stimuli require only minimal processing at the structural level before analysis begins at the semantic level, thereby reducing the response time to such a stimulus because of an element of predictability. Such a system would be compatible with the distinction between **controlled** and

**automatic** systems of information processing proposed by Shiffrin and Schneider (1977).

Schneider, Dumais and Shiffrin (1984) propose that 'certain types of memory modification may be largely a control-processing function' (p. 2). Controlled processing of memory (encoding) is limited in its capacity, being slow and serial in nature (occurring one step at a time). They suggest that any form of memory modification must transcend the controlled information processing stage if it is likely to stand a chance of becoming consolidated as an automatic method of encoding and retrieval.

IDENTIFYING DISORDERS OF ATTENTION

Deficits in attention and concentration are often unrecognized by psychologists because standard cognitive tests, or the neuropsychological measures conventionally used in clinical practice, rarely focus upon attention itself even though there is an implicit assumption that attention is a necessary process for good performance on these tasks. Newcombe (1985) states that such tests 'rarely tap the patient's capacity to focus and shift attention' (p. 159). She feels that even behavioural tests of attention yield ambiguous information and quotes Hink and Hillyard (1978) who suggest 'one cannot ascertain whether the data reflect selective attention . . . or general attentiveness . . . or both' (p. 159). Reasons for this apparent dislocation between subjective experience and objective test data lie in an understanding of the interaction between attention and cognition, and the failure of standardized neuropsychological or cognitive tests to elicit information which reflects this relationship. Mateer and Sohlberg (1986, 1988) consider the problems of using conventional tests to assess attention. They divide clinical measures of attentional capacity into four broad categories.

1. Tests that primarily assess immediate or working memory
2. Tests in which performance on simple information processing is timed
3. Tests in which information provided per time unit is controlled or 'paced'

4. Tests that incorporate information processing in the face of high or low level distraction.

They point out that these tests are very different in the requirements placed on a patient and, as a group, fit no consistent conceptual model. Clinical assessment of memory they feel, rarely, if ever, reflects information that explains the relationship between attention, information processing, and memory. As an example they cite the studies by Harris and Wilkins (1984) and Wilkins and Baddeley (1978) on prospective memory. This is the type of memory problem most commonly described by patients (e.g. forgetting appointments or the content of telephone calls) and most closely linked to attentional difficulties, especially reduced attentional capacity.

The ability of an individual to perform well on a diverse number of tasks depends not simply on having sufficient cognitive ability to understand the tasks *per se*, but upon an ability to focus and maintain attention during the task and simultaneously, an ability to divide attention *across* those tasks. During the performance of any one task, an awareness has to be maintained of the presence of other tasks which may need to be completed according to certain priorities of time, or in terms of economy of effort (implying organization). In real-life situations, for example, many behaviours need to occur concurrently if 'performance' is to be maintained. The inability to divide attention has been used as a basis for explaining a number of accidents (Reason, 1984).

In an earlier edition of this volume, Wood (1984) introduced some concepts from academic psychology to try and explain how components of attention can be considered as important to the learning capabilities of a brain-injured person receiving rehabilitation. These components of attention (arousal, selectivity and effort) can now be further sub-divided according to their clinical manifestation which represent various **disorders of attention**.

## DISORDERS OF AROUSAL

Arousal is 'the ability to be awakened, to maintain wakefulness, and to follow signals and commands'. (Stuss and

Benson 1986, p. 98). It represents one component of an 'orienting response' (Sokolov, 1963) which itself is important to maintaining a level of awareness and necessary for preserving the state of consciousness (Eames and Wood, 1984). Arousal therefore, is an important mechanism helping to maintain a level of **alertness** of an organism.

The clinical manifestation of disorders of arousal or alertness are quite varied, ranging from higher level disorders of arousal where responsiveness is consistent but slow ('obtundation'), to the lowest level of arousal or non-responsiveness, when the disorder is described as **coma**. Somewhere in between, but probably not on the same continuum, is the clinical phenomenon of **akinetic mutism** (Cairns 1952) which involves sleep-wake cycles, but little observable cognitive or motor functioning. Stuss and Benson (1986) describe this as a 'striking example of an attention-arousal disorder' (p. 98).

Benson and Geschwind (1975) describe the phenomenon of 'drifting attention' which occurs in cases of focal pathology to the brain stem reticular activating system. Patients in this condition can attend to a stimulus (e.g. the therapist) for brief periods of time but a disorder of (tonic) alertness, results in only a transient level of attention being maintained. As a result, the patient frequently returns to an under-aroused or somnolent state. More common are the complaints of patients who have sustained mild or moderate concussional injuries who, when attempting to read or watch television, just 'drift-off' and become pre-occupied with other ideas, leading to a distraction from the main activity.

In cases where damage to the arousal component of attention is implicated, disorders of drive are a common legacy. Individuals who have sustained serious frontal injury, or those where diffuse cerebral injury is suspected (following anoxia) frequently display a behaviour pattern which is dominated by a lack of activity, interest, initiative and perseverance (Eames and Wood, 1984). Such patients invariably appear to be under-aroused (under-alerted) and show a tendency to drowsiness and somnolence. This has been referred to as a disorder of drive and has poor prognostic implications for patients receiving rehabilitation following brain injury (Wood, 1987; Eames and Wood, 1984).

Individuals may appear lethargic and apathetic and seem incapable of translating ideas into action.

Disorders of drive should not be confused with feelings of fatigue. Fatigue is probably one of the most universal complaints after head injury. Feelings of exhaustion often follow periods of activity which normally would be taken in one's stride. Superficially, this may be attributed to physical exertion, yet, 'the most common complaint, even amongst individuals whose work and life habits are much more physical than intellectual, is that it is **mental activity** which most readily induces fatigue' (Eames and Wood, 1984, p. 10).

The difference between a disorder of drive and a feeling of fatigue is that fatigue almost always occurs following some kind of effort, whereas a reduction in drive prevents an individual making such an effort and is often seen in association with a loss of initiative and spontaneity. Disorders of drive therefore have serious implications for those aspects of behaviour which involve motivation. Wood (1987) discusses how a reduction in drive can interfere with an individual's ability to recognize or appreciate (and respond to) various forms of cognitive reinforcement and can even prevent an individual reacting in a clinically beneficial way to various forms of encouragement or reinforcement (even the more controversial and ethically dubious methods of behaviour modification, e.g. punishment).

## DISORDERS OF SELECTIVE ATTENTION

The process of selective attention is one in which an individual **selectively attends** to certain environmental stimuli in preference to others (Kahneman, 1973, p. 3). The process can be broadly sub-divided on the basis of the kind of activity in which the individual is engaged. Some activities require **focused** attention, while others require attention to be **divided** over several objects or sets of stimuli. In either case the object of the exercise is to avoid being distracted by events which are peripheral or unimportant to on-going behaviour.

Focused attention is more commonly identified with selective attention because it requires attention to be centred on one kind of information in preference to (and to the exclusion of) other sources of information. Divided attention on the other hand requires a level of awareness which is broad enough to be divided, or shared, between two or more sources or kinds of information, or two or more mental operations. The classical example of focused attention is the 'cocktail party phenomenon' in which a guest tries to listen to one conversation and ignore all others.

An inability to maintain a focus of attention is one of the most common disorders of attention following concussional injury. Patients report that they cannot watch television, or read a newspaper, if somebody is talking in the background. This is the phenomenon most commonly referred to as distractibility (as defined as a failure to focus attention and inhibit external **noise**). Distractibility can be attributed to a deficit in conscious, directed, attentive **behaviour**. Stuss and Benson (1986) attribute this to a disorder of the fronto-thalamic gating system, failing to regulate responses to environmental stimuli.

### DISORDERS OF EFFORT AND INFORMATION PROCESSING

'Effort' emphasizes the **control process** of attention Posner and Boies (1971); McGuinness and Pribram (1980); Stevens (1981). This control process co-ordinates alertness, arousal and selectivity, in order to maintain an adequate level of awareness and direct attention towards significant features of the environment. This aspect of attention is most frequently referred to as **'concentration'** and, as such, it is clearly a very important component of attention, one which is vital to the learning process. It is this aspect of attention which appears particularly vulnerable to the effects of brain injury.

Kahneman (1973) suggested that processing resources (**effort**) are mobilized in response to task demands and that there is a fixed allocation of effort for each task. Time pressure, which is inherent in the structure of most tasks, increases processing demands. In Kahneman's words, 'Investment of less than this standard effort causes a deterioration of performance, but in most tasks it is impossible to eliminate errors completely by a voluntary increase in effort.

Davis (1983) stated that our information processing ability

is dependent upon several factors. First we depend upon the quality of stimulus input; the more obvious the stimulus, the less effort is needed to 'search' for it. Secondly we depend upon the availability of mental structures to perform the cognitive operations necessary for processing the input. Finally we require a mental capability to provide the energy required for those cognitive operations to be carried out.

Clearly, the third component is critical to the way an individual deals with the information available in his environment. The mental resources have been assumed to be allocated to the mental structures involved in the processing of information but the capacity of the brain to do this is determined by control processes which form part of, or are linked to, the memory system and in which attention is either equated with momentary capacity or non-specific mental effort (Kahneman, 1973; Davis, 1983).

## REHABILITATING ATTENTION DISORDERS

Until recently, relatively little work has been directed at rehabilitating disorders of attention. To some extent this can be attributed to the lack of a clear understanding about the nature of the attention process and its central importance as a mediator of many other aspects of cognitive behaviour, including memory.

The rehabilitation of attention can be broadly divided into two areas. The first involves attention as a form of behaviour. This includes **attentiveness**, roughly defined as directing head and eyes towards an object or activity, but also includes responding to environmental stimuli which act as important cues to guide or direct human behaviour. The second broad area of attention training incorporates cognitive components of attention and should perhaps be referred to as improving the information processing capability of the brain. This aspect of attention training would appear to have great significance for therapists involved in the rehabilitation of memory disorders because it deals with the primary system by which information is passed into and out of memory (Atkinson and Shiffrin, 1968). The following sections will attempt to review and evaluate some of the work that has been carried out on attentional retraining in these two areas.

IMPROVING ATTENTIVENESS

**Attentiveness** is a form of behaviour that is required for a diverse number of activities, (e.g.)

1. Sustaining attention for the purpose of participating in therapy tasks
2. Recognizing and responding to changes in environmental conditions
3. Visual scanning; possibly in cases where visual field deficits prevail.


INCREASING SUSTAINED ATTENTION

Problems of short attention span were recognized as early as 1904 when Kulman proposed that they could explain the learning difficulty experienced by mentally handicapped people. Strauss and Kephart (1947) considered short attention span to be the main problem underlying the difficulty that brain injured children displayed attending to task for any length of time and learning new skills. More recently, psychologists and others who work with the brain injured have become increasingly aware of the role of this aspect of attention as a factor influencing learning in rehabilitation.

Possibly one of the first aims of attention training is to improve an individual's capacity to sustain attention. This helps reduce the effects of distractibility, improves concentration during therapy sessions, facilitates co-operation between patient and therapist and thereby provides the patient with a better opportunity to learn new techniques.

It is important to provide training in sustained attention in both visual and auditory modalities. Initially, each modality should be trained separately, but when task performance has improved to an acceptable level, both modalities can be combined increasing the demands of the attention task and increasing the realistic nature of the procedure (most forms of social behaviour require bi-modal attentional monitoring).

In the first volume of this book 'vigilance training' was described as a method for increasing attention span and improving concentration. The method required a patient to monitor a sequence of auditory or visual information and respond to pre-determined targets which occurred at random intervals over a 30- or 60-minute period. Although it is an essentially boring procedure it has proven an effective method of improving both the behavioural components of attention as well as increasing the information processing capabilities of the patient.

Recently, Wood (1986) has described a method of behavioural training, using a fixed interval schedule of reinforcement which allows therapists systematically to reward patients for maintaining an attentional set and **attending to task** during rehabilitation activities. This procedure is relatively easy to administer and can be applied in a variety of rehabilitation therapies where 1:1 patient-therapist interactions take place. This system of increasing the **effort** component of attention has now been successfully applied to a number of patients with different types of brain injury of varying degrees of severity and at different stages in recovery, with uniformly successful results. There are indications that the procedure generalizes from the training task to other therapy activities that are not directly included in the training programme.

These aspects of attentive behaviour are all dependent upon sustained attention which incorporates the concept of **effort** referred to above.

RECOGNIZING AND RESPONDING TO ENVIRONMENTAL CUES

Human behaviour relies upon an ability to recognize changes in the environment that have implications for regulating our actions or determining the nature of on-going behaviour (see Wood, 1990 a and b). Environmental 'cues' may take various forms. They can be as diverse as sudden changes in speed or position of vehicles on a motorway, indicating that changes may have to take place in our driving behaviour in order safely to negotiate potential motorway hazards. Alternatively, we may need to modify our social behaviour in circumstances when the feedback we receive from others suggests that our comments or style of behaviour is inappropriate, e.g. telling a rude joke in the presence of people who find such comments embarrassing!

Human behaviour is therefore based on a continual appraisal of the feedback we receive from our interaction with the environment. Shallice (1982) suggested an information processing model called the **supervisory attentional system (SAS)** which monitors specific or routine aspects of behaviour that can be activated by any form of mental activity. Shallice refers to a procedure he described as **'contention scheduling'** which quickly selects actions in response to the strongest perceptual triggers. This system of contention scheduling therefore controls which environmental stimuli will be selectively attended to.

The model proposed by Shallice is highly complex but has an intuitive or common-sense appeal. In order to make optimal adjustments to our behaviour we need to know what to look for in our environment, and this means being able to focus our attention on relevant cues which act as feedback for the regulation and organization of behaviour, simultaneously ignoring aspects of our environment which provides feedback that may be irrelevant to on-going behaviour. This procedure implies a form of **discriminative attention**. Wood (1987, 1988a) showed how the ability to **recognize** what is important in terms of feedback from the environment is extremely important, even to the most basic forms of learning. Discriminative attention was seriously impaired in people who had sustained severe brain injury and significantly interfered with their ability to respond accurately on a simple discrimination learning task. This deficiency was found to be relatively independent of intelligence meaning that individuals with an average or even high IQ could lack the essential discriminative qualities of perception that allowed them to recognize, and respond to, relevant cues in their environment. Consequently, there was an inevitable failure on the part of these individuals to organize and plan actions, or acquire simple skills based on discrimination learning procedures. These forms of cognitive deficit were almost invariably predominant in individuals who had sustained serious frontal lobe damage.

REMEDIATING DISCRIMINATIVE ATTENTION

A relatively simple example of how a failure of discriminative attention can interfere with routine aspects of behaviour was seen in a 23-year-old girl who had sustained a severe head injury with post-traumatic amnesia in excess of two months. In addition to bilateral cortical damage she had also sustained a mild brain-stem injury and was dependent upon a wheelchair for mobility.

Progress in rehabilitation was complicated by a number of factors, not least her inability to focus and sustain attention. Gradually, she acquired the ability to feed herself, and could wash and dress with only minimal supervision. The aim of the rehabilitation was to help this young woman reach a stage of independence where supervised residential care in the community was appropriate. The day hospital programme that she was attending had achieved most of the rehabilitation objectives but the ability to train the patient in independent toilet transfers (from wheelchair to toilet) had consistently eluded them.

A functional analysis of the skills that comprised this transfer ability indicated that the patient was not making appropriate use of environmental cues in order to position her wheelchair in such a way that would allow her to complete the transfer movement fluently and without danger of falling. Once this problem was recognized an attempt was made to provide a **prosthetic environment** by using brightly coloured sticky tape to help her position her wheelchair correctly, initially at the door of the bathroom, and later, adjacent to the toilet, at a point where a successful transfer could be made.

At first, the bright red tape was used in abundance, in order to help the patient attend to and recognize the salient cues, allowing her to position her wheelchair appropriately. Once reliable positioning and successful transfers had been established, the amount of tape was systematically reduced until gradually it was removed altogether, leaving only the 'normal' environmental cues to guide behaviour. The reduction of cues took place without any deterioration in the transfer skill. The procedure, which is similar to the method of 'errorless learning' proposed by Cullen (1968), shows how manipulating attentional factors in the environment allowed the successful establishment of a safe and reliable transfer movement making it possible for the patient to be discharged into an appropriate residential setting.

ESTABLISHING HABIT SEQUENCES OF BEHAVIOUR

In an elegantly written chapter, Reason (1984) reminds us of the historical emphasis based on the attentional regulation of behaviour. He quotes James (1890) who referred to the fact that, 'habit diminishes the conscious attention with which our acts are performed' (p. 114). Reason, in his discussion on the role of habit as a regulator of behaviour, refers to attention as 'the gate-keeper to consciousness' (p. 156). He considers both habit and attention to play a leading part in the guidance of behaviour and there is a clear overlap between the nomenclature used by Reason (1984), Shiffrin and Schneider (1977) and Shallice (1982). They all refer to the fact that attention is involved in behaviour to different degrees depending upon the level of skill that has been attained.

In a new task, for example, one needs to pay close attention to the consequences of one's action in order to achieve certain goals (Reason, 1984). With increasing practice, however, the sequence of actions or behaviours becomes more automatic and requires less conscious attention. Some 'action sequences' can become so fluent and automatic that giving too much attention can actually disrupt the smooth flow of motor output (e.g., such as trying to think about where to place one's feet when running up or down stairs – a form of cognitive interference over an automatic motor sequence that almost inevitably precipitates a fall).

A possible problem for rehabilitation therapists is that too much of human behaviour exists at an automatic level. Some of the basic requirements for independent living all feature as automatic action sequences, e.g. putting food to one's mouth; getting washed; dressed; walking, etc. In many cases of serious brain injury, these automatic behaviours are disabled and patients have to revert to a conscious mode of behaviour which requires a major adjustment to the way we think about behaviour.

For many individuals the major obstacle preventing the restoration of independence is not physical disability but the loss of basic automatic **action sequences** which need to be established at a more conscious and regulated attentional level. This problem will be easily recognized by nurses and therapists who regularly encounter the kind of individual who is physically able but cognitively disabled, to the point that he needs close support and supervision to perform relatively simple and routine self-care skills. Wood (1987) gave a number of examples of individuals who are not able to learn how to wash or dress, not because of physical disability, but because of some form of cognitive impairment. The training methods to overcome this handicap were described in the context of behaviour modification procedures. These procedures employ basic principles of learning in an attempt to obviate many of the cognitive deficiencies preventing such individuals re-acquiring skills that promote functional independence.

Perhaps the cognitive basis of this behavioural training to re-establish habit sequences of behaviour can be explained in the following case history.

A 35-year-old male suffered a severe concussional head injury when a truck tyre, which he was inflating, exploded in his face, throwing him several feet into the air. He sustained a basilar skull fracture and bilateral frontal contusions with a right fronto-parietal subdural haematoma. He remained in coma for several weeks with a post-traumatic amnesia of at least three months. His neurological recovery was unremarkable and he was more or less physically intact, but he displayed major neuropsychological legacies of this injury, including perseveration of ideas, confabulation, grandiose thinking, information processing difficulties combined with an inability to focus and sustain his attention.

The process of getting this patient washed and dressed each morning was quite laborious. His behaviour was extremely disorganized and, if left on his own, he would take an inordinate time to dress (almost invariably without washing) and the pattern of his behaviour would be fragmented, undirected and essentially without any purpose.

In order to establish a more productive sequence of behaviour that led to greater self-care in washing and dressing, the complex response pattern that comprised this aspect of his behaviour was broken down into 23 units of activity. Initially, each unit of activity was prompted by a member of the staff at the Transitional Living Centre in which the patient was a resident. At first, the patient did not reliably respond to each prompt and several prompts might be required before an appropriate response was obtained allowing the next unit of behaviour to take place. Gradually, the patient acquired a reliable response pattern to these individual prompts, allowing the 23 units of behaviour to be condensed into 12 larger response sequences, each one preceded by one prompt which presented the patient with more information and required a much greater and more complex response.

This procedure successfully trained the patient to complete the complex action sequence with only a minimal number of prompts. As training progressed, the patient was observed to connect automatically one unit of action with another, therefore displaying a more spontaneous sequence of behaviour, initiating activities in a logical sequence yet (apparently) without consciously (or cognitively) attending to the behavioural process itself. Through this form of behavioural training (shaping a complex behaviour pattern by chaining together individual units of the activity) staff were able to bypass or reduce the cognitive demands that such a learning procedure might otherwise have required. It is interesting to note that this habit sequence was maintained even in the absence of the structure provided by the transitional living centre because the behaviour was maintained at weekends and other holiday periods when the patient returned to his family home.

## VISUAL SCANNING TRAINING

The inability to recognize and respond to environmental cues is often based upon a failure to scan one's environment effectively. Many forms of brain injury result in disorders of visual scanning and this has been proposed as the main goal of rehabilitation in cases of visual neglect and hemi-inattention (Diller and Weinberg, 1977; Weinberg, Diller, Gordon *et al.*, 1977). They consider visual scanning deficiencies to have implications for a variety of functional skills that lead to independence and the quality of outcome following brain injury rehabilitation.

The remediation of visual scanning employs a procedure which is broadly based on behavioural learning strategies combining procedures which rely on attention and information processing abilities. Diller and Weinberg maintain that the task of training patients to compensate for hemi-inattention and poor visual scanning is to present tasks that are sufficiently compelling in order for patients to feel motivated to direct attention towards them. Next it becomes necessary to guide the patient's scanning in a directed and regulated search of their environment, providing them with cues to assist in systematic and orderly scanning. As the patient improves, these cues are gradually reduced to allow the patient to perform the activity spontaneously.

A training apparatus described as a 'scanning machine' was used to help patients co-ordinate visual scanning ability. The machine incorporates two rows of ten coloured lights with a target light that traverses the perimeter of the board. The activation of each light is controlled by the cognitive therapist and the patient is expected to monitor the movement of the light by pointing to it as it travels around the edge of the board. Initially, a patient's head movements are slow and 'jerky' as they attempt to follow the target but with practice the head movement becomes regulated with increased fluency of visual scanning, following the target smoothly at varying speeds, regardless of whether the target moves in a right to left or left to right direction.

Diller and Weinberg describe this process in a behaviourally oriented way and there is clearly an overlap between many of the assumptions underlying this procedure and those described previously with respect to training self-help skills. The experience of Diller and his colleagues suggests that much of the disability seen in hemi-inattention and related visual scanning deficiencies is due to a faulty set of 'habits' that co-exist with neuropsychological disabilities. By forcing individuals to view stimuli systematically and repeat the training procedures that have become automatic, they have been able to train these individuals to compensate for hemi-inattention.

## REHABILITATING THE CONTENT OF ATTENTION

The disturbances of attention described above interfere with the channelling of information into awareness. The content of mind would therefore seem to depend upon how much information is channelled into awareness and the organization of that information in terms of its significance to the organism. In many ways, this is the basis of the memory system, as the previous comments on 'working memory' (Baddeley and Hitch, 1974) propose. Anything that interferes with the reliable storage of information will reduce the content of awareness and have serious implications for memory.

It must be emphasized that there is a fundamental relationship between attention and memory with a dependence of the latter upon the former. Nissen (1986) stated that 'information that is not attended to is poorly remembered' (p. 17). Craik and Lockhart (1972) propose that an event was more likely to be remembered if it achieved a deeper level of processing than an event that was only processed briefly or superficially. It would appear, therefore, that a major aim of attentional training should be to achieve a level of information processing that actually translates into greater understanding, better awareness and a more reliable memory.

Unfortunately, there is little evidence to show that we can influence the **content of attention**. Wood (1986) found that patients who made significant progress on attention training tasks, improving aspects of (a) attention span, (b) discriminated visual processing, and (c) speed of response, failed to generalize that ability to other tasks that call for good information processing in verbal and auditory modalities.

### COMPUTER TRAINING PROCEDURES

The computer revolution in cognitive rehabilitation has modulated slightly since its introduction during the early 1980s as a panacea for all cognitive ills! In fairness, there is a *prima facie* case for thinking that the information processing requirements involved in many computer games or tasks might have a general influence on cognitive functioning, leading to greater awareness and better organizational thinking.

The early claims for computer rehabilitation techniques made by Bracy (1983), Lynch (1983) and Trexler (1982) have not been supported by more systematic or controlled evaluation procedures. Bracy claimed to have used computer training procedures to improve intelligence test scores in three patients who were three years post-injury. No attempts were made to control for spontaneous recovery and it is interesting to note that the sub-test scores which have the highest attentional loading (e.g. digit symbol test) showed no improvement over the period of training. Lynch (1983) gave examples of using conventional computer games (e.g. space invaders) to improve aspects of information processing but there is no evidence that the progress made by individuals on these tests generalized to other aspects of behaviour or improved the content of awareness and memory in any way.

More recently, controlled studies by Ponsford and Kinsella (1988) employing a multiple baseline design to evaluate a computer training procedure for the remediation of deficits in speed of information processing, failed to produce any clinically viable results. They administered a three-week training programme to ten severely head injured subjects at an average interval of 13.8 weeks post injury. Training tasks were selected to provide repeated practice in responding rapidly, but selectively, to visual information presented on a computer screen. The progress of the experimental group was compared to a control group consisting of 16 orthopaedically injured patients. Ponsford and Kinsella found that once spontaneous recovery and practice effect were controlled, there was no significant difference between the two groups in their response to the computer training procedures.

Another control study was completed by Wood and Fussey (1988) using 20 severely brain-injured patients, all of whom were more than two years post-injury. The training procedure was based on a task which required focused attention, discriminative perception, selective judgement, visual scanning, and response speed. Pre- and post-training measures were obtained using tests which demanded good visuomotor ability and visual memory. The performance of ten patients in the computer training group was compared with ten controlled patients, matched for severity of brain injury, sex and level of intelligence. All the patients in the training group showed a significant improvement by reducing their error rate on the computer task and increasing speed of information processing. However, post-test measures on the related visual memory and visuo-motor tasks showed that there was no evidence of any generalization to these modality-related tasks and, once practice effect had been controlled for, there was no difference between the training and control group on the outcome measures.

## SUMMARY

Attentional processes represent a complex fabric that connect and integrate a number of cognitive functions, co-ordinating the flow of information throughout the brain in such a way that intellectual **ability** becomes translated into intellectual **activity**. This chapter has attempted to show that disorders of attention can have an adverse affect on all cognitive skills and interfere with many aspects of behaviour. If rehabilitation therapists ignore the role of attention as a mediator of awareness, influencing the ability of individuals to understand and respond to salient aspects of the environment, opportunities may be lost for improving the learning potential of individuals receiving therapy because the demands of the rehabilitation activities exceed the attentional processing capabilities of the patient.

Improving attention would appear to be an important prerequisite for any form of cognitive rehabilitation and should also be considered as a preliminary to many other forms of rehabilitative therapy. Clinical studies have now shown that it is possible to increase aspects of sustained attention, improving the learning opportunities of the patient because improved **concentration** usually implies improved **co-operation**.

So far, most of the advances made in attentional retraining have been at the behavioural level of attention (attentiveness and visual scanning). These modest achievements should not be under-estimated because they can be used to improve a number of activities of daily living, as the earlier clinical examples demonstrate. These achievements also indicate that cognitive retraining should not be considered in narrow terms, neither should it rely too heavily on computer technology. Computers are a relevant part of cognitive rehabilitation but their potential is still unclear and appears limited, relative to the opportunities offered by cognitive-behaviour procedures. It is anticipated that the greatest success in cognitive retraining will come from improving the ability of patients to focus and sustain attention on relevant aspects of their environment while modifying their behaviour in response to changing environmental situations.

## REFERENCES

Atkinson, R.C. and Shiffrin, R.M. (1968) Human Memory: A proposed system and its control processes; in K.W. Spence and J.G. Spence (eds), *The Psychology of Learning and Motivation*, 2 Academic Press, New York, 97–123.

Baddeley, A.D. and Hitch, G.J. (1974) Working Memory; in G.A. Bower (ed), *The Psychology of Learning and Motivation*, 8, Academic Press, New York.

Baron, A., Myerson, J. and Hale, S. (1988). An integrated analysis of structure and function of behaviour. In G. Davey and C. Cullen (eds.) *Human Operant Conditioning and Behaviour Modification* Wiley, Chichester.

Benson, D.F. and Geschwind, N. (1975) Psychiatric conditions associated with focal lesions of the central nervous system. In *American Handbook of Psychiatry, Vol. 4: Organic Disorders and Psychosomatic Medicine*, 2nd ed, edited by S. Arieti and M. Reiser, 208–43, Basic Books, New York.

Bracy, O.L. (1983) Computer based cognitive rehabilitation. *Cognitive Rehabilitation*, 1, 7–9.

Cairns, H. (1952). Disturbances of consciousness with lesions of the brain and diencephalon. *Brain*, 75, 109–46.

Caveness, W.F. (1969) Post-traumatic sequelae. In A.E. Walker, W.F. Caveness and M. Critchley (eds) *The Late Effects of Head Injury*, Springfield, Ill: Charles C Thomas, 209–19.

Conkey, R.C. (1938) Psychological changes associated with head injuries, *Archives of Psychology*, 232, 1–62.

Craik, F.I.M. and Lockhart, R.S. (1972) Levels of processing: A framework for memory research. *Journal of Verbal Learning and Verbal Behaviour*, 11, 671–84.

Craik, F.I.M. and Tulving, E. (1975) Depth of processing and the retention of words in episodic memory. *Journal of Experimental Psychology*, 104 (3), 268–94.

Cullen, C.N. (1968) Errorless learning with the retarded, *Journal of Practical Approach to Development of Handicap*, II, 21–4.

Davis, D.R. (1983) Attention, arousal and effort, In, A. Gale and J.A. Edwards (eds.) *Physiological Correlates of Behaviour*, Vol. 2, Academic Press, London, 9–30.

Denker, S.J. and Lovfring, B. (1958) A psychometric study of identical twins discordant for closed head injury, *Acta Psychiatrica, Neurological Scandinavia*, **33**, Suppl. 122.

Diller, L. and Weinberg, J. (1977) Hemi-attention in rehabilitation: The evolution of a rational remediation program. In E.A. Weinstein and R.P. Freidland (eds). *Advances in Neurology*, New York, Raven Press, **18**, 63–82.

Eames, P.G. and Wood, R. Ll. (1984) Consciousness in the brain damaged adult, In R. Stevens (ed). *Aspects of Consciousness*, **4**, Academic Press, London 1–35.

Geschwind, N. (1982) Disorders of attention: A frontier in neuropsychology. In, D. E. Broadbent and L. Weiscrantz (Eds) *The Neuropsychology of Function*. London, Royal Society, 173–85.

Goldstein, K. (1939) *The Organism*, American Book Company, New York.

Harris, J.E. and Wilkins, A.J. (1984) Remembering to do things: A forgotten topic: In J.E. Harris and P.E. Morris (Eds). *Everyday memory actions and absent mindedness*. New York: Academic Press, 97–115.

Hecaen, H. and Albert, M.L. (1978) Human Neuropsychology. John Wiley and Sons, New York.

Hink, R.F. and Hillyard, S.A. (1978) Electrophysiological measures of attentional processes in man as related to the study of schizophrenia. *Psychiatry Research*, **14**. 155–65.

James, W. (1890) *The Principles of Psychology*. New York, Holt.

Kahneman, D. (1973) *Attention and Effort*. Englewood Cliffs, N.J., Prentice-Hall.

Kulman, E. (1904) Experimental studies in mental deficiency. *American Journal of Psychology*, **15**, 391–446.

Lezak, M.D. (1983) *Neuropsychological Assessment*. New York, Oxford University Press.

Lockhart, R.S., Craik, F.M. and Jacoby, L. (1976) Depth of processing, recognition and recall. In J. Brown (ed.) *Recall and Recognition*. John Wiley and Sons, Bath.

Lynch, W. (1983). Cognitive retraining using microcomputer games and commercially available software. *Cognitive Rehabilitation*. **1** (1), 19–22.

Mahoney, M.J. (1974) *Cognition and Behaviour Modification*. Ballenger, Cambridge, Mass.

Mateer, C.A. and Sohlberg, M.M. (1986) *Efficiency of Attention and Prospective Memory Training*. Unpublished paper presented at the University of Victoria Neuropsychology Workshop, Victoria, B.C.

Mateer, C.A. and Sohlberg, M.M. (1988). A paradigm shift in memory rehabilitation. In *Principles and Practices of Cognitive Rehabilitation*. Guilford Press.

Mateer, C. A., Sohlberg, M. M. and Crinean (1987) Perceptions of memory function in individuals with closed head injury. *Journal of Head Trauma Rehabilitation*, **2**, 74–84.

McGuinness, D. and Pribram K. (1980) The neuropsychology of attention: emotional and motivational controls. In M. Whitlock (ed.), *The Brain and Psychology*, New York, Academic Press, 256–82.

References 241

Meyer, A. (1904) The anatomical facts and clinical varieties of traumatic insanity. *American Journal of Insanity*. **60**, 373–441.

Morris, P. (1978) Encoding and retrieval, In *Aspects of Memory*, (ed) M.M.Gruneberg and P. Morris, London, Methuen, 61–84.

Newcombe, F. (1985) Neuropsychology of consciousness: A review of human clinical evidence. In, A.D. Oakley (ed.), *Brain and Mind*, Methuen, London, 152–97.

Nissen, N. J. (1986) Neuropsychology of attention and memory. *Journal of Head Trauma Rehabilitation*. **1** (3), 22–31.

Ponsford, J. and Kinsella, G. (1988) Evaluation of a programme for attention deficits following head injuries. *Journal of Clinical and Experimental Psychology*, **10**, 639–798.

Posner, N. and Boies, S. J. (1971) Components of attention, *Psychological Review*, **78**, 391–408.

Reason, J. (1984) Lapses of attention in everyday life. In R. Parasuraman, (ed.) *Varieties of Attention*, Academic Press. London, 515–50.

Ruesch, J. (1944) Intellectual impairment in head injuries, *American Journal of Psychiatry*, **100**, 180–96.

Shallice, T. (1982) Specific impairment in planning. In D. Broadbent and L. Weiskrantz (eds.) *The Neuropsychology of Cognitive Function*. The Royal Society. London, 285–304.

Schneider, W., Dumais, S. T. and Shiffrin R. M. (1984) Automatic and control processing and attention. In R. Parasuraman (ed.), *Varieties of Attention*. Academic Press, London.

Shiffrin, R. M. and Schneider, W. (1977) Controlled and automatic human information processing. II, perceptual learning, automatic attending and a general theory. *Psychological Review*, **84**, 127–90.

Sokolov, Y.N. (1963) Perception and the conditioned reflex. *Ann. Review, Physiol.* **25**, 545–80.

Stevens, R. (1981) Brain mechanisms and selective attention. In G. Underwood and R. Stephens (eds.), *Aspects of Conciousness, Vol.* **4**, *Clinical Issues*. Academic Press. London.

Strauss, A. and Kephart, N. (1947) *Psychopathology and Education of the Brain Injured*. New York: Grune and Stratton.

Stuss, D.T. and Benson, D.F. (1986) *The Frontal Lobes*, Raven Press, New York.

Teasdale, G. and Mendelow, D. (1984) Pathophysiology of head injuries. In D.N. Brooks (ed.) *Closed Head Injury: Psychological, Social and Family Consequences*. Oxford Medical Publications, 4–36.

Trexler, L. (1982) *Cognitive Rehabilitation, Conceptualization and Intervention*. Clennan Press, New York.

Underwood, G. (1978) Attentional activity and behaviour control. In G. Underwood (ed.) *Strategies of Information Processing*. Academic Press, London, 193–225.

Weinberg, J., Diller, L., Gordon, W. A. *et al.* (1977) Visual scanning training effect in reading-related to tasks in acquired right brain damage. *Archives of Physical Medical Rehabilitation*. **58**, 479–86.

Wilkins, A. and Baddeley, A. (1978) Remembering to recall in everyday life: An approach to absentmindedness. In, M. Gruneberg, P. Morris and R. Sykes (eds.). *Practical Aspects of Memory*. New York, Academic Press.

Wood, R.Ll. (1984). Management of attention disorders following brain injury. In B.A. Wilson and N. Moffat (eds.). *Clinical Management of Memory Problems*. Croom Helm, London.

Wood, R.Ll. (1986). Rehabilitation of Patients with Disorders of Attention. *Journal of Head Trauma Rehabilitation*. 1 (3), 43–53.

Wood, R.Ll. (1987) *Brain Injury Rehabilitation: A Neurobehavioural Approach*. Croom Helm, London.

Wood, R.Ll. (1988a) Attention disorders in brain injury rehabilitation. *Journal of Learning Disabilities*, **21**, 327–33.

Wood, R.Ll. (1988b) The management of behaviour disorders in a day treatment setting. *Journal of Head Trauma Rehabilitation*, (3), 53–62.

Wood, R.Ll. (1990a) Towards a Model of Cognitive Rehabilitation. In *Cognitive Rehabilitation in Perspective*, R. Ll. Wood and I. Fussey (eds), Taylor and Francis, London.

Wood, R.Ll. (1990b) Neurobehavioural Paradigm for Brain Injury Rehabilitation. In *Neurobehavioural Sequelae of Traumatic Brain Injury*, R.Ll. Wood (ed.) Taylor and Francis, London.

Wood, R. Ll. and Fussey, I. (1988). Computer-based cognitive retraining: A controlled study. *International Disability Studies*. **9**, 149–53.

# Chapter 9

# The development of group memory therapy

## BARBARA WILSON AND NICK MOFFAT

Therapists are invariably short of time, and one way of dealing with this situation is to treat people in groups rather than singly. A more important reason for working with groups rather than individuals is the possibility that memory-impaired people may benefit from interaction with others having similar disabilities. Many memory impaired people believe they are losing their sanity, and this fear may be alleviated by observing others with similar difficulties. Participants in a group may also give advice to each other and may be more likely to use aids or strategies if their peers are seen to be using them. The influence of a peer group on an individual's behaviour is likely to be stronger than the exhortations of a therapist, however well intentioned the latter may be. It has also been observed that memory groups have face validity: participants (and their relatives) believe that treatment given in groups is effective, and this in itself may have indirect therapeutic value. Furthermore, it is nearly always possible to ensure that each member of a group succeeds at something during a meeting because group therapy provides such a wide range of tasks of varying difficulty. For people used to failure it is no bad thing to provide an element of success in front of their peers. Finally, given our current level of knowledge, running a memory group is probably educational for the therapist. Considerable information can be gained by noting different patients' responses to different strategies: we can learn, for instance, which tasks are enjoyed by most patients and which are not; and we can record the occurrence of particular problems for certain members of a group and subsequently adopt alternative approaches.

This chapter will be divided into four main parts. First,

the literature on memory groups will be reviewed. Second, the evaluation of the Rivermead Memory Group will be described. Third, the development of memory groups which are run in East Dorset will be outlined. Finally, issues in organizing and evaluating a memory group will be discussed.

REVIEW OF LITERATURE ON MEMORY GROUPS

This review will be divided into three sections, covering group treatments for different types of client.

First, the earliest research on group therapy, which evaluated classroom or formal reality orientation training for patients with dementia, will be discussed. Second, group therapy for people without obvious organic impairment but who complain of memory problems will be considered. Finally, memory groups for people with memory problems resulting from, for example head injury, stroke or excessive use of alcohol will be described.

**Classroom or formal Reality Orientation training**

Reality Orientation (RO) was first described by Dr James Folsom, (Folsom, 1967, 1968) as a rehabilitation technique to meet the sensory and emotional needs of long-stay elderly psychiatric patients (see Moffat, this volume). More recently RO has been concerned with helping the elderly confused patient, particularly to improve cognitive and behavioural functioning.

The two main means of achieving this have been informal RO (also known as 24-hour RO), and formal RO (also known as classroom RO or RO groups).

Formal RO sessions were initially considered to be a supplement to informal RO but increasingly have been used in isolation. Sessions may be held five days a week for half-an-hour each day, with a group leader and three to six persons according to the level of confusion. In a basic group, emphasis will be placed upon the presentation and repetition of current information and the provision of prompts and reinforcement. For those who are less confused, an advanced group can be formed which will have higher expectations regarding orientation, and group members may be able to engage in more extended discussions.

### Formal RO versus control treatment condition

Of the five main studies comparing formal RO sessions with a control condition, three reported beneficial effects, whilst two found a detrimental effect.

First, Brook, Degun and Mather (1975) compared formal RO sessions with exposure to the RO room but without active therapist participation. The authors observed significant improvement only in the behaviour of the group with an active RO therapist.

A more adequate control for level of staff involvement was available in the studies by Voelkel (1978) and MacDonald and Settin (1978), who compared RO with a resocialization group and a sheltered workshop respectively. In both studies the results were unfavourable to RO. Thus, Voelkel's resocialization group improved more than the RO group on the orientation test. However, two factors should be considered in interpreting these results. First, the resocialization group contained activities similar to those used by others in their RO sessions, suggesting that the two treatments were not that dissimilar. Second, the two groups were not adequately matched, with the RO groups being initially more impaired. This may have been of significance because in most of the RO studies, with the exception of Hanley's (1981) ward orientation training, the less severely impaired patients improved most.

An important consideration in both the Voelkel and the MacDonald and Settin studies was the matching of the style of training to the level of functioning of the patients. Both studies reported that some patients found RO sessions irritating and childlike. This may help to explain why MacDonald and Settin (1978) found that the sheltered workshop group, who made gifts for residents in a nearby school, showed significant improvements on a self-report life satisfaction index, whilst the RO group showed a non-significant decline in life satisfaction over the same time period. In this study there were no changes in observer-rated behaviour following either the five week formal RO sessions, or a similar time spent in the sheltered workshop activities.

The fourth controlled study, reported by Woods (1979), found general deterioration in the rated behaviour of the patients, regardless of whether they were in the RO or social therapy groups, or in the no-treatment control. However, there was some evidence in favour of the RO group. Thus, compared with the social therapy and controls, the RO group showed a significant improvement on tests of information, orientation and on the learning of complex and novel information from the Wechsler Memory Scale (Holden and Woods, 1982). Generally, the staff were more enthusiastic about the social therapy than the RO sessions, indicating a more than adequate control for staff attention. There was some suggestion that the social therapy group actually showed greater deterioration on measures of concentration than the RO or control group. Unfortunately, the small sample size of four or five patients in each condition makes it difficult to interpret these results, particularly as many studies have commented on the wide range of individual responsiveness to treatment.

A modified version of formal RO was devised by Hart and Fleming (1985), which incorporated social and material reinforcement and shaping procedures (limited recognition tasks) in the therapy sessions. As predicted, they found that this modified formal approach, with its greater reliance upon established learning theory principles, produced greater increase in orientation than the matched control group receiving the traditional formal RO relying primarily upon rehearsal. However, neither group resulted in generalization observed (time sampled) talking outside the therapy sessions. Furthermore, at the eight-week follow-up period both groups had returned to baseline levels on the orientation measures. The interpretation of this study suffers from two major limitations. First, the patients had varied diagnoses, with more schizophrenics having a longer length of hospitalization in the traditional RO groups. Second, traditional RO had been in existence on the wards for eighteen months before the introduction of the modified approach. Therefore, the limits of the value of RO therapy for these patients may have already been achieved. Nevertheless, the modified approach may have generated increased interest and willingness to participate, even if it did cause additional frustration for one patient.

### Formal RO or individual RO versus no treatment

Overall, there have been some encouraging results from the studies which have provided formal RO, indicating that something is better than nothing. Improvements in verbal orientation have been noted by most authors, Johnson, McLaren and McPherson (1981), Goldstein *et al.* (1982), Greene (1984) and Hanley (1986). Even the one study which did not find a significant improvement in orientation following RO training at least noted a weak trend in favour of RO (Hogstel, 1979). However, with regard to generalization of formal RO to other behaviours, the results are more mixed.

First, there are reports of no behavioural changes, as noted by Holden and Sinebruchow (1978), Hanley *et al.* (1981) and Goldstein *et al.* (1982).

Second, there are reports of generalization which are derived from poorly controlled studies. For example, Holden and Sinebruchow (1979) reported behavioural improvement and increased scores on the Holden Communication Scale. Unfortunately, this study not only contained a mixed group of patients, but may have included some use of the informal 24-hour approach. Perhaps more importantly, the results appear to indicate that all of the patients improved regardless of their participation in the RO sessions. Another example is the thinly described study by Merchant and Saxby (1981) which does not present adequate data to support the claim of increased ability to hold a conversation and increased awareness of others.

Third, there are reports of no generalization of training. For example, the group cross-over design of Goldstein *et al.* (1982) found similar results to the individual training described by Woods (1983). Both studies reported improvements on trained items, with no generalization to untrained but similar orientation items. Furthermore, Goldstein *et al.* (1982) reported no generalization to ward behaviour, but overall noted wide individual differences in response to the RO training.

Finally, one study which does offer very encouraging results is that by Greene, Timbury, Smith and Gardner (1983). This was carried out in a psychogeriatric day hospital with twenty dementia patients using a group ABA design. Formal RO training was given two or three times a week for six weeks. This resulted in a significant improvement on the personalized orientation test, and the Clifton Assessment Schedule. As predicted, the benefits relapsed after the RO training ceased. The ingenious feature of the Greene *et al.* (1983) study was that the relatives completed ratings of the patient's behaviour, and of their own mood and stress, whilst being blind to the presence of a reality-orientation-training phase during the weeks of monitoring. The relatives reported a significant improvement in the mood of the patient following RO training, which again relapsed after treatment ceased. However, there were no systematic changes in other aspects of the patient's behaviour. In particular it was noted that the relatives reported a significant improvement in their mood following the RO phase, with slight reductions also being noted in feelings of personal distress and negative feelings towards the patient. The mood of the relative appeared to relapse again following cessation of reality orientation training.

Greene *et al.* (1983) report that the improvements followed a predictable temporal sequence with improvements in orientation preceding those on the Clifton, and improvements in the patient's mood preceding those in the relative. Although this is an encouraging study in demonstrating generalization of training, it contains inherent weaknesses. First, other forms of interaction might have had an equivalent effect upon the patient and the relative. Thus, an adequate control condition needs to be established in future research of this kind. Second, as with some other RO studies (Hanley, 1981; Woods, 1983; McCartney, 1984; and Hanley, 1986), the possibility of relapse has been exploited to strengthen the ABA experimental design. However, from a clinical point of view it would be important to maintain treatment gains and to research the factors which might be necessary in order to maintain any initial gains (Rusch and Kazdin, 1981).

The Greene *et al.* study demonstrated improvements in both the patient's and relatives' mood when a formal reality orientation group was provided for the patient. However, when the relative was involved in the therapy group for the patient, the results were less encouraging, especially for the relative. Thus, Zarit, Zarit and Reever (1982) worked with dementia sufferers and their carers, who were randomly allocated to one of three conditions, a didactic group providing training in visual imagery, a problem solving group dealing with everyday memory difficulties, or a waiting-list control. It was found that more of the patients in the didactic and problem-solving groups than in the waiting-list condition improved or stayed the same on recall but not recognition memory measures. The relatives attending the didactic and problem-solving groups became more depressed, perhaps because of a growing awareness of the level of impairment of their dependants. It may be that the people with dementia were too impaired to be able to benefit from memory training (Yesavage, 1982) and even if they were able to do so, the technique may be of limited value to the person and the family. However, there was some indication that the problem-solving group was of some practical help since there was a non-significant reduction in reported memory and behaviour problems, and there was a tendency for the relatives to be less distressed when the problems did occur. Perhaps shorter meetings instead of one and half hour sessions might be more appropriate for dementia sufferers. Furthermore, a longer course, instead of seven meetings over three and a half weeks, would result in a greater opportunity to put into practice the ideas generated within the group.

Thus, overall there is generally favourable evidence for formal RO sessions with confused elderly patients. However, this statement requires qualifying because, as has been described above:

1. changes have been only slight, with limited generalization to other cognitive or behavioural measures;
2. there have been some negative outcomes following formal RO;
3. formal RO has sometimes been compared only with no treatment and so the specific benefits of RO relative to other stimulation procedures cannot be established.

## Memory groups for people without amnesia

Memory therapy need not be confined to helping patients with obvious memory impairment. Healthy people may have a desire to improve their memory performance, and certainly some elderly people who might be particularly anxious or depressed and complain of concentration or memory problems would benefit from memory group work.

In a study involving non-confused elderly subjects Zarit (1979) found that an interpersonal skills group was equally as effective as a memory skills group in improving memory performance and reducing memory complaints. Zarit also showed that a current events group and a waiting list were ineffective at altering memory performance, but that the current events group did result in reduced memory complaints. Thus, following participation in any of the groups, subjects reported a reduction in memory complaints. A factor which may have contributed to this was that subjects were screened before participation and only those with no cognitive impairment were able to participate in the study. This in itself may have reassured those subjects who might have volunteered because of a concern about their memory ability.

Higbee (1981) found that students who took a memory-improvement course showed improvements in recall of a word list, and also a lasting positive change in self-perception of memory ability. However, the students did not continue to use the memory techniques, and in line with other studies of the use of study techniques, the memory course did not result in improvements in college grades (Gadzella *et al.*, 1987).

## Memory groups with amnesic people

In the first edition of this book (Wilson and Moffat, 1984) the memory groups run by each of the authors for their respective brain-injured patients were described. Wilson had developed and run the Rivermead Memory Group, whilst Moffat had started the Birmingham Memory Group. The groups we described differed slightly in terms of format and content, but there was a common aim of teaching memory strategies, the carrying out of group memory exercises and the completion of home practice. At that time no other memory groups were known to exist, and no evaluations had been completed. In subsequent years a number of people have run memory groups, although only one evaluation has been reported.

Godfrey and Knight (1985) randomly allocated twelve hospitalized alcoholic amnesics to either memory therapy or control treatment of non-specific activation. The sessions were held four times a week for eight weeks and evaluation consisted of laboratory-based memory tests, practical tasks and ratings by nurses (the In-patient Memory Impairment Scale, Knight and Godfrey, 1984). The memory group practised four types of task: associate learning using slides of visual material, picture recognition, recalling a trip made around the hospital and reality orientation exercises. The results indicated that regardless of whether the subjects were in the memory group or the non-specific activation group, they showed the same level of improvement on most measures, including those that assessed generalization of memory skills.

Thus, in accordance with some of the evaluations of formal RO mentioned earlier, the study by Godfrey and Knight (1985) found non-specific effects of participation in group therapy but not specific improvements in memory performance compared with controls.

The need for controlled evaluation of memory groups was also recognized in the evaluation of the Rivermead memory group which compared three weeks of daily memory training with an equivalent amount of time for problem solving.

## RIVERMEAD MEMORY GROUP

An evaluation of the Rivermead Memory Group was carried out with the assistance of Zafra Cooper and Helen Kennerley.

### Subjects

Subjects were selected from in-patients at Rivermead Rehabilitation Centre. Those who met the following criteria were

**Table 9.1** Evaluation of the Rivermead memory group

| Weeks | Cohort A (N=9) | Cohort B (N=11) |
|---|---|---|
| 1 & 2 | 2 pre-treatment assessments | 2 pre-treatment assessments |
| 3,4,5 | memory group | problem-solving group |
| 6 | intermediate assessment | intermediate assessment |
| 7,8,9 | problem-solving group | memory group |
| 10 | post treatment assessment | post treatment assessment |
| 1 year | follow-up | follow-up |

chosen from within a group of patients referred to the clinical psychology department for help with memory problems:

1. subjects whose scores on at least one of the memory tests fell in the impaired range, and
2. whose condition remained stable (spontaneous improvement being absent).

Of 25 patients referred, 22 met the criteria. Two of these were discharged before completing treatment thus leaving 20 patients in the study. There were 12 men and 8 women, with a mean age of 31.9 years (SD 15, range 13–63). Fifteen had received a very severe head injury which was followed by unconsciousness for ten days or more. The mean length of coma for these patients was 6.4 weeks (S.D. 6.1 weeks, range 10 days to 6 months). Four patients had suffered a cerebral vascular accident and one was post encephalitic. The mean length of time post insult was 10.25 months (SD 9.8 months, range 2–36 months). The mean Full Scale IQ was 91.3 (SD 14.4, range 73–133). Performance IQs tended to be lower, the mean being 81.7 (SD 17.7, range 54–131).

### Assessment procedures

The following tests were administered in order to measure memory functioning.

*Standardized tests*

1. Prose recall – immediate and delayed. Passages were taken from the Wechsler Memory Scale (1945). Stories from the

WMS were used in the following order: first assessment – first story from Form 1; second assessment – second story from Form 1; third assessment – first story from Form 2; fourth assessment – second story from Form 2. For the follow-up one year later the first story from Form 1 was used again.

2. Digit Span – forwards and backwards digit span tasks from the WMS were used with different versions at each assessment.

3. Paired Associate Learning – the Randt *et al.* (1980) paired associates were employed. There are four alternative versions of this test in which six pairs of words are selected, four of them having a semantic association (e.g. 'card'-'board') and two pairs having no obvious associations (e.g. 'corn'-'map'). Three trials were given on each occasion. At one year follow-up the first version was re-administered. The maximum score for each administration was 18.

## Behavioural measures

1. The Rivermead Behavioural Memory Test (Wilson, Cockburn and Baddeley, 1985) was administered during each assessment. The test uses tasks analogous to those encountered in normal everyday living (e.g. remembering an appointment, remembering to deliver a message, learning a new route). There are twelve items in the test, each is scored pass/fail, resulting in a possible maximum score of twelve. Versions A, B, C and D were administered in order, with version A readministered at the one-year follow-up.

2. The adapted Kapur and Pearson (1983) rating scale was administered on three occasions (once prior to treatment, once at the end of treatment and once at the one-year follow-up). It was not administered during the intermediate assessment due to shortage of time. In retrospect, however, this measure would have been useful. Scores range from 0 to 20, with a low score indicating the subject believes s/he has many severe problems.

3. An adapted version of Harris' (1980a) questionnaire on the use of memory aids was given on the same occasions

as the rating scale described above. There is one score for each aid used and a maximum score of twelve.

## Treatment procedures

Training in the Memory Group involved the following six stages.

1. Playing memory games and practising various memory exercises (e.g. Kim's Game and Pelmanism);
2. Group discussion of problem-solving techniques (e.g. asking how a member of the group coped with a particular memory difficulty);
3. Introducing external memory aids (e.g. notebooks, electronic aids);
4. Practice in using external aids;
5. Introducing internal strategies (e.g. visual imagery and mnemonics);
6. Practice in using internal strategies.

The problem-solving group was designed to be as much like the memory group as possible but without introducing any special techniques for improving or exercising memory. Obviously it was not possible to avoid memory tasks altogether as memory is involved in all but the most reflex activity. The tasks selected for the problem-solving group included both verbal and non-verbal tasks taken from a variety of sources. These included the following:

1. *The Five-Day Course in Thinking* (De Bono, 1979);
2. *Raven's Progressive Matrices* (Raven, 1960);
3. *Luria's Neuropsychological Investigation* (Christensen, 1975);
4. *Games of Logic* (Berloquin, 1980);
5. *Evans' Attainment Tests* (Wing and West, 1973);
6. A series of tests devised by the therapists at Rivermead (e.g. making up as many words as possible from the word 'rehabilitation').

## Results

The study was concerned with five main questions, each of which will be considered in turn:

1. Was there a difference between the two cohorts of subjects prior to treatment with regard to their memory deficits?

   A series of t-tests was used to look at differences between Groups A and B prior to treatment. No significant differences were found on any of the measures of memory impairment, with the exception of paired associate learning. Here there was a difference in favour of the second assessment ($t = 4.14$ d.f. $= 19$). In the absence of change on any other measures between the first and second pre-treatment assessments the most likely reason for better scores on the second administration of paired associate learning is that the pairs in Form 2 of the test are easier to learn.

2. What changes, if any, occurred in memory functioning following treatment?

   The mean scores pre- and post-treatment, and at one year follow-up can be seen in Table 9.2. Given that no differences were obtained between the two pre-treatment measures (with the exception of paired associate learning), the second of the two pre-treatment measures was used as a comparison with the immediate post-treatment measure. This decision was taken in order to reduce any effects in cases where minor and non-significant natural recovery was taking place.

   A series of analyses of variance was applied to the data and provided the following results:

   (a) There was a significant improvement in the RBMT scores following treatment ($F = 6.7$, d.f. 3, 57, p $<0.001$). A Newman-Keuls Test indicated that there was a significant difference in RBMT scores following both memory group and problem-solving group training. Although memory group training led to more improvement, the difference between the two kinds of group was not significant. There was also a significant difference between pre-treatment and follow-up scores, although not between post-treatment and follow-up.

   (b) There was also a significant difference in the immediate logical memory scores ($F = 3.55$, d.f. 3, 57, p $<0.05$). However, a Newman-Keuls Test showed that

**Table 9.2** Mean scores of all subjects pre- and post-treatment and at follow-up

| TEST | PRE-TREATMENT | POST-MEMORY GROUP | POST PROBLEM-SOLVING GROUP | ONE YEAR FOLLOW-UP |
|------|------|------|------|------|
| RBMT | 2.75 | 4.95 | 4.15 | 4.85 |
| ILM | 5.30 | 6.35 | 5.55 | 7.15 |
| DLM | 1.30 | 1.70 | 1.80 | 2.85 |
| P-As | 10.00 | 10.85 | 11.00 | 12.20 |
| DF | 6.40 | 6.35 | 6.80 | 6.20 |
| DB | 4.15 | 4.10 | 4.20 | 4.15 |

RBMT = Rivermead Behavioural Memory Test
ILM = Immediate Logical Memory
DLM = Delayed Logical Memory
P-A's = Paired Associates
DF = Digits Forward
DB = Digits Backward

the only difference here was between the follow-up scores and the pre-treatment scores. (The passage used at follow-up was the same as that used at the first pre-treatment assessment.)

(c) Similar results were found on the delayed logical memory scores ($F = 2.73$, d.f. 3, 57, $p < 0.05$). Again, the Newman-Keuls Test showed that the only significant difference was between the pre-treatment and the one year follow-up scores.

(d) With regard to paired associate learning, the results are more complex. Because of the pre-treatment differences both sets of pre-treatment scores were included in the analysis of variance. There were significant differences between the sets of scores ($F = 14$, d.f. 4, 75, $p < 0.001$). As with the logical memory scores, the one year follow-up scores were better than pre-treatment scores ($p < 0.01$), but in this case post-treatment scores were better than the first pre-treatment scores and *not* better than the second pre-treatment scores.

(e) With both digits forwards and backwards no significant differences emerged on any occasion. (For digits forwards $F = 1.7$, and for digits backwards $F = 1.49$. In both cases d.f. $= 3 + 57$.)

**Table 9.3a** Scores of individual patients on the RBMT and self-report rating scale of memory difficulties.

### A. PRE-TREATMENT

```
GOOD
MEMORY   12
         11
         10
          9
          8         *
          7    *
          6    *            *
          5  *              *
          4       *         *      *
          3     *
          2       *
BAD       1                *
MEMORY    0  * * * *        *     *    **
             0 1 2 3 4 5 6 7 8 9 10 11 12 13 14 15 16 17 18 19 20
             MILD                 RATING SCALE            SEVERE
```

### B. POST-TREATMENT

```
GOOD
MEMORY   12
         11
         10  *              *
          9
          8        *    *
          7        * *       **
          6  *  *            *
          5     *
          4        *
          3     *
          2
BAD       1  *  *                    *
MEMORY    0           *        *
             0 1 2 3 4 5 6 7 8 9 10 11 12 13 14 15 16 17 18 19 20
             MILD                 RATING SCALE            SEVERE
```

3. Were patients aware of their memory impairments and did awareness improve with treatment?

A series of product moment correlations was carried out between patients' ratings of their memory failures and their scores on the RBMT. If patients were able to judge accurately the severity of their memory deficits then a significant negative correlation would be expected, as a

**Table 9.3b** Scores of individual patients on the RBMT and self-report rating scale of memory difficulties

```
                   C. ONE YEAR FOLLOW-UP
GOOD
MEMORY     12  *
           11
           10
            9             *  *
            8
            7   *   *   * *   *    *          *
            6                  *
            5   *
            4       *
            3           *
            2
BAD         1   *       *
MEMORY      0  *     *       *
               0 1 2 3 4 5 6 7 8 9 10  11  12  13  14  15  16  17  18  19  20
MILD                       RATING SCALE                          SEVERE
```

*Mean scores of all subjects pre and post treatment and at follow-up*

| Test | Pre-treatment | Post Memory Group | Post problem-Solving group | One year Follow-up |
|------|---------------|-------------------|----------------------------|--------------------|
| RBMT | 2.75  | 4.95  | 4.15  | 4.85  |
| ILM  | 5.30  | 6.35  | 5.55  | 7.15  |
| DLM  | 1.30  | 1.70  | 1.80  | 2.85  |
| P-As | 10.00 | 10.85 | 11.00 | 12.20 |
| DF   | 6.40  | 6.35  | 6.80  | 6.20  |
| DB   | 4.15  | 4.10  | 4.20  | 4.15  |

RBMT = Rivermead Behavioural Memory Test
ILM = Immediate Logical Memory
DLM = Delayed Logical Memory
P-A's = Paired Associates

high rating score indicates many problems while a high RBMT score indicates few everyday memory failures. No significant correlations were obtained at pre-treatment (r = −0.13), post-treatment (r = −0.16), or at follow-up (r = −0.13). However, some individuals did appear to have reasonable insight into the nature and severity of their problems, as can be seen from Table 9.3. It can also be seen that others had no idea at all of the severity of their impairment. There was a tendency for patients to *underestimate* the severity but not to *overestimate*.

An analysis of variance comparing rating scales at pre- and post-assessments and one year follow-up showed no evidence of change in ratings over time (F = 1.65, d.f. 2, 34).

4. Did the use of memory aids increase as a result of treatment?

Analysis of variance showed a significant difference in the number of memory aids reported (F = 13.9, d.f. 2, 34, p <0.01). A Newman-Keuls Test showed that a significantly higher number were used at the one year follow-up in comparison with pre-treatment (p <0.01) and with post-treatment (p <0.01), although there was not a difference between pre- and post-treatment findings. No direct observations were made to see whether these aids were in fact used. Table 9.4 summarizes all the ANOVA results.

5. Was it possible to determine which patients were likely to respond favourably to treatment?

No obvious pattern emerged to suggest which patients were likely to respond best to treatment. Neither time post insult nor age would appear to be important. A comparison of the six patients who showed greater over-all change with the six who showed least change revealed no significant difference in mean time post insult. There was a difference in mean age (28.33 compared with 37.83

**Table 9.4** F ratios from summary of ANOVA results
(Pre- and Post-treatment and follow-up)

| TEST | DF | F RATIO | P VALUE |
|---|---|---|---|
| RBMT | 0, 57 | 5.7 | 0.001 |
| IMMEDIATE LOGICAL MEMORY | 3, 57 | 3.55 | 0.05 |
| DELAYED LOGICAL MEMORY | 3, 57 | 2.73 | 0.05 |
| PAIRED ASSOCIATE LEARNING | 4, 76 | 14.00 | 0.001 |
| DIGITS FORWARDS | 3, 57 | 1.7 | N.S. |
| DIGITS BACKWARDS | 3, 57 | 1.49 | N.S. |
| RATING SCALES | 2, 34 | 1.65 | N.S. |
| USE OF MEMORY AIDS | 2, 34 | 13.90 | 0.01 |

**Table 9.5** A comparison of the ages (in years) and the time post insult (in months) of the six subjects who responded best and the six subjects who responded worst to treatment

|  | AGES (Years) | | TIME POST INSULT (Months) | |
|---|---|---|---|---|
|  | BEST | WORST | BEST | WORST |
|  | 28 | 39 | 5 | 10 |
|  | 21 | 19 | 10 | 2 |
|  | 39 | 38 | 11 | 35 |
|  | 27 | 62 | 5 | 3 |
|  | 42 | 27 | 5 | 4 |
|  | 13 | 42 | 8 | 2 |
| MEAN: | 28.33 | 37.83 | 7.33 | 9.33 |

years). However, the large variability in age and the small sample size make it difficult to draw firm conclusions from this finding. Table 9.5 shows the individual ages and the time post insult from the six best and the six worst responders to treatment.

The picture becomes no clearer at the one year follow-up. On the RBMT, for example, six people scored better at follow-up than post-treatment, six scored worse, and eight showed no change. Although the mean ages, time post insult, length of coma and IQ score differ to some extent for each group, as can be seen in Table 9.6, there is nevertheless considerable overlap.

Although the mean length of coma and mean time post insult are longer for those who deteriorated, the differences are not significant (F = 1.13, d.f. 2, 13, and F = 1.1, d.f. 2, 17 respectively)

### Conclusions

Overall, the results of the evaluation of the Rivermead Memory group are consistent with the majority of studies described earlier; e.g. Godfrey and Knight (1985), Zarit (1979), and Zarit, Zarit and Reever (1982), which found that there were no specific benefits of a memory group compared with a matched control condition.

However, these studies do provide some important implications for the development of memory groups.

**Table 9.6** Characteristics of subjects at the one year follow-up

|  | IMPROVED (N=6) | SUBJECTS STAYED THE SAME (N=8) | DETERIO-RATED (N=6) |
|---|---|---|---|
| NO. OF HI'S | 5 | 5 | 5 |
| MEAN AGE FOR ALL Ss | 24.5 | 39.8 | 28.6 |
| MEAN LENGTH OF COMA FOR H.I.'s (weeks) | 5.1 | 4.5 | 9.7 |
| MEAN TIME POST INSULT (months) | 9.5 | 7.2 | 15.1 |
| MEAN VIQ | 96.8 | 91.8 | 108.8 |
| MEAN PIQ | 78 | 75 | 92.8 |
| MEAN FSIQ | 88.4 | 83.7 | 102.5 |

First, in general a structured group is at least better than nothing (e.g. Zarit, Zarit and Reever, 1982).

Second, where differences in outcome do occur they are generally in the predicted direction, in that the greater the structure of the group the better the outcome. Thus, reality orientation was found to be superior to social therapy (Woods, 1979), and a modified form of reality orientation training was superior to traditional reality orientation (Hart and Fleming, 1985). Third, it is important that the tasks in the group are appropriate for the level of ability of the participants. Thus, tasks may be too easy and boring, such as basic reality orientation with patients who do not have generalized memory and intellectual impairment (McDonald and Settin, 1978; Voelkel, 1978). On the other hand tasks may be too demanding, such as the use of visual imagery with patients who have dementia (Yesavage, 1985).

Fourth, tasks and strategies should be directly applicable to the everyday needs of the person. Thus, under conditions such as where the strategies are aimed at coping with everyday memory problems or where particular strategies are taught, use of memory strategies may be maintained for at least one month after the completion of a group (Hermann et al., 1988). This is an improvement over the more usual problem of people not maintaining use of the various strategies which have been taught in memory classes (Cornoldi, 1988; Higbee, 1981; Lapp, 1983).

Fifth, measures of outcome following participation in a memory group or control treatment need to be sensitive to the small changes in memory performance which may occur, and broad enough to detect any improvements from amongst the varied types of memory (which may not relate closely to one another). This may explain why, in the memory group evaluation described above, the Rivermead Behavioural Memory Test was sensitive to participation in a group whilst more specific tests were not. Furthermore, as Cornoldi (1988) suggests, the effects of training may not be limited to memory improvements, since the subjects' increased confidence in their memory abilities (see Higbee, 1981) 'may extend this positive attitude to other problems to be faced'. Thus, the significant improvements in the patient's mood and then the mood of the relative in the Greene *et al.* (1983) study involving reality orientation training is worth replicating, particularly if a control treatment is also provided.

In recognition of the issues raised above, the next section of this chapter will describe the present format of the East Dorset Memory Group. This group is now quite different from the group which had been run by the same author in Birmingham (Wilson and Moffat, 1984), and outcome measures are being developed which, it is hoped, will be more sensitive to the kinds of improvement which participants had reported.

### DEVELOPMENT OF THE EAST DORSET MEMORY GROUP

The Memory Group in East Dorset is an outpatient group which has evolved from the original group run in Birmingham (Wilson and Moffat, 1984). The present group meets weekly for ten weeks, followed by three follow-up sessions at monthly intervals. The group size has varied from four to ten, together with two therapists (the author and usually a trainee clinical psychologist or psychology technician).

The participants have been recruited from routine referrals to the author for assessment and/or rehabilitation. The participants have had varying levels of amnesia and aetiologies,

**Table 9.7** Content of memory group sessions

| WEEK | TOPIC |
|------|-------|
| 1 | How my memory works |
| 2 | Making the best use of my memory |
| 3 | Making remembering easy |
| 4 | Concentrating |
| 5 | Practice makes perfect |
| 6 | Remembering to do things |
| 7 | Remembering information such as the News |
| 8 | Listening and expressing an idea |
| 9 | Tackling other problems |
| 10 | Continuing to use memory techniques |

but an important consideration has been that the person has some insight into the problems.

It appears that the most successful groups have included members with similar problems (e.g. people recovering from a head injury), whereas a more heterogeneous group which includes members who have progressive conditions, alongside those who are recovering from a head injury, have generally been less successful. Each group session lasts for one hour, which includes a short tea break. Handouts, which include home practice assignments, are provided each week. The programme for the ten sessions of the group is listed in Table 9.7 and described in more detail below.

A description of each session follows.

### Session 1 – 'How my memory works'

Exercises are carried out during the group session (and as home practice assignments) which illustrate the types of memory (see Baddeley, 1983), and which test the ability of the participants accurately to judge their own performance on different types of memory task.

### Session 2 – 'Making the best use of my memory'

This session focuses upon the relationship between mood and memory performance (or more especially the perception of memory performance). This is discussed with regard to anxiety, depression, good and bad days, and confidence levels. Training in relaxation and self-instructions is provided in order to help cope with memory tasks and when lapses of memory have occurred.

### Session 3 – 'Making remembering easier'

Four main types of external memory aid are discussed:
Temporary storage (e.g. notebooks and shopping lists);
Long-term storage (e.g. encyclopaedias and address books);
Forward planner (e.g. diary and calendar);
Environmental changes (e.g. keeping things in a special place).

The use of these memory aids is encouraged, particularly as they may be infrequently used (Wilson and Moffat, 1984b) or their value may be under-estimated (Leng *et al.*, 1988).

### Session 4 – Concentrating

Various ways in which concentration can be disrupted are discussed and ways of maintaining concentration are outlined. These include: Concentrating over time (e.g. incorporating brief rest periods when reading);
Overcoming external distractions (e.g. work in a study or quiet room and doing one thing at a time);
Overcoming internal distractions (e.g. using self instructions to deal with intrusive thoughts).

### Session 5 – Practice makes perfect

Each group member identifies information to be learned, such as people's names or items of general knowledge. One new item is selected for practice each day using prepared work sheets. Practice of that item is spaced out during the day using a rule of doubling the time interval in between practice sessions (e.g. practice of an item occurs at 10.00 a.m., 10.02, 10.04, 10.08, approximately 10.15, 10.30, 11.00 a.m., 12 noon, 2.00 p.m., 4.00 p.m., and then the next day). More details of this procedure are provided in Moffat (this volume).

### Session 6 – Remembering to do things

The separation of remembering to do things from other types of memory is described, and personal examples of successes and failures on this kind of task are elicited. Methods for helping to reduce the chances of forgetting to do things are outlined and home practice assignments at this kind of task are agreed.

### Session 7 – Remembering information

The story recall procedure (PQRST, Glasgow *et al.*, 1977) is described and then practised using short newspaper articles (see Moffat, this volume, for more details of this technique). Home practice includes the application of this procedure to written articles and then to the television news using prepared worksheets.

### Session 8 – Active listening and expressing an idea

Written guidelines are provided on cards to help group members improve their listening skills and expressive ability. The guidelines incorporate some of the study techniques practised in the previous week. Group exercises include each member presenting a topic to the group. Cards are also issued to group members which they can give to other people so that they can help group members to keep pace with a conversation and retain the main points of what has been said.

### Session 9 – Tackling other problems

The many and varied concerns of group members are shared, including other cognitive problems, and emotional, family, financial or legal problems. Specific help is provided during the group session, via home-based practice or by additional sessions if required.

### Session 10 – Continuing to use memory therapy techniques

Ways are sought to help group members maintain and increase the application of the strategies learned during the group. This includes revising particular sessions on set dates and making reminders of particular strategies (e.g. a bookmark with the PQRST study technique written on it). Tasks are set which are to be completed by the follow-up session.

### ORGANIZING AND EVALUATING A MEMORY GROUP

Some of the difficulties encountered in running a memory group will be similar to those found in organizing any kind of group: selecting appropriate group members; finding a suitable time and place for meetings; uncertainty about how much leadership to provide; concern about how best to organize the activities and how much general discussion to encourage or control. Our intention is to concentrate on issues specifically relating to memory groups, which seem to us to have a particular set of problems that are in many ways different from those experienced by other kinds of groups involved in rehabilitation.

### Membership

Before starting a new group it is necessary to consider the particular needs of each individual to ensure that the final grouping has a reasonable chance of achieving some degree of success. At this initial stage it is quite possible that some individuals will be excluded because their problems are not only different from the majority of the group but they may also cause a conflict of interests within the group. Others will be saved embarrassment by exclusion from the group. An intelligent person with a classic amnesic syndrome and no other deficits may be unwilling to co-operate in a group which contains a confused, disturbed, physically handicapped, head-injured person and a disinhibited frontally damaged patient. People who have right hemisphere damage and non-verbal memory problems but whose verbal memory is above average may not believe there is anything the matter with them. Furthermore, they may feel affronted by being placed in a group with people who cannot remember anything that was said to them two minutes earlier. Ideally, some degree of homogeneity is desirable.

We exclude people who have severe speech or language problems, partly because we feel they will be embarrassed at not being able to communicate freely in our groups and partly because most of the group exercises involve speaking and comprehending. Nevertheless, mild aphasics have been included at times and they have participated fully and with obvious enjoyment. Others excluded from the group are those with severe behaviour problems because they are so disruptive. This is not to say that people with such problems should not be included in a group at all but simply to point out that their disruptive behaviour may make progress within a memory group impossible. Patients who are severely and generally intellectually impaired are also excluded. To participate in the group it is necessary to have reasonable comprehension and motivation. Most of the group members are able to read and write – at least to an eight- or nine-year-old level.

There is little point in running the memory group if fewer than four patients are present. On certain days, there will be absentees through sickness or other pressing appointments within the unit. Ideally, there should be two members of staff available to run the group session. This ensures that memory group sessions can be run continuously even though one or other of the leaders may not be available on certain days. However, it would be undesirable to have too broad a spectrum of staff members involved in the organization of the memory group as continuity and cohesion might suffer.

### Practical Issues

Members may need reminders to attend. e.g. a telephone call the morning of the group, and transport arranged so that they do not get lost. Those making their own way to the group may arrive at incorrect times (wrong time of day or incorrect day), and allowance has to be made for early, or more usually, late, arrivals. It can be helpful to have other group members provide a synopsis of what has been discussed for the benefit of the late arrival. Time will be required for re-capping on what has taken place in previous sessions and extra copies of handouts available for those who have lost them.

In addition, group members usually find it difficult to concentrate in the group and to remember what is being said. Therefore, it is important to use a quiet room, which has a large board or flip chart so that information can be written down to remind members what has happened so far and what is planned for the remainder of the session. The inclusion of a tea break in the middle of each session helps to maintain concentration by dividing the session into two short time periods.

## Management

In managing a memory group the leader has to be aware of the wide variety of needs of individual patients. As mentioned earlier, ensuring some degree of success is one of the principles of a memory group and working on a problem-free area is one way of achieving this. Other ways of obtaining successful outcomes may involve some engineering of the time interval. Most participants will have an adequate immediate memory span, so asking one of them to do something immediately will increase the chances of success. Those with a less severe impairment can be asked after a long delay. Similarly, in the reality orientation exercises the easiest question for most people is 'What year is it now?' This question can be asked of the most disoriented person, at least on some occasions. For patients who find almost every task too difficult we include some motor memory activities, for example, tracking tasks or reaction-time tasks. Improvements on these can be almost guaranteed even though the patient may not remember having completed them before. These improvements should, of course, be charted or recorded in some way so that feedback of success can be provided. Audio or video recordings are alternative ways of providing feedback of successful performance which would not normally be remembered by patients.

Group members are encouraged to talk about memory problems which have recently occurred or situations they are about to face so that practical advice can be offered. Reports on successes are strongly encouraged to enhance individual and group morale.

There will be other patients in the group who will spend too little time on their areas of greatest need. If possible, some individual memory therapy should be provided for these. Failing this, it may be necessary to set the rest of the group a task which they can do on their own while the group leader spends time attending to the needs of a particular individual. Alternatively, when both leaders are in attendance one of them can work with an individual for some of the time.

Another potentially difficult area concerns the relationships that exist between patients. The behaviour of one patient may cause a disturbance among others. The group might include a person who will not stop talking (a fairly common difficulty after head injury) and who never gives anyone else a chance to answer a question or raise a point; or there may be a person who quarrels incessantly with everyone, or who sees himself as superior to the group and consequently refuses to participate. There are no easy answers to the problems raised by such patients. In some cases ignoring the disruptive behaviour might be the wisest solution, while for others an explanation about the effects they have on the rest of the group might be effective. Possibly a formal behaviour modification programme to reduce the problem behaviours might lead to the most effective changes.

## Evaluation

As has been described earlier, there have been very few reports on the effects of memory training provided in groups, and hence it is too early to draw any firm conclusions about the efficacy of memory groups. There appear to be three main issues which need to be addressed in future research: improving the process of therapy; improving the measures of outcome; and providing an adequate control group.

### Improving the process of therapy

First, tasks need to be selected which match the ability level of the patient since, in some studies, tasks have proved to be either too easy (e.g. McDonald and Settin, 1978) or too difficult (e.g. Yesavage, 1982). Furthermore, future research should investigate the structure of the training, since in general the greater the structure the greater the benefit (e.g. Hart and Fleming, 1985). This will only be detected if the measures for evaluating outcome are appropriately selected and, if necessary, developed.

## Improving the Measures of Outcome

Given that the evaluations so far have reported only modest changes in memory performance, measures need to be sensitive to change. This can be achieved by use of a broad-based test battery such as the Rivermead Behavioural Memory Test, or by the use of a number of specific tasks. A comprehensive evaluation should include the use of memory strategies and the level of subjective memory complaints as reported by the amnesic person, and also a relative. In addition, measures need to be included (or developed) which assess the person's mood and ability to cope with memory problems.

It can also be beneficial to assess the mood of the relative, since this can be enhanced by the person's participation in a group (Greene *et al.*, 1983) or be adversely affected (Zarit *et al.*, 1982).

Some of the measures which have been suggested above are currently being piloted as part of the East Dorset Memory Group (e.g. assessment of mood, and coping with memory problems).

## Provision of control group

In order to control for non-specific effects it is important to provide an adequate control group. It would also be worthwhile looking at any subjects who do respond to the memory group or else to the control conditions, so that a clearer indication of the appropriate selection criteria can be determined.

Present studies of group memory therapy have illustrated some of the problems and limitations of existing approaches. The challenge for future studies will be to develop efficacious and cost-effective means of helping people with memory problems.

## REFERENCES

Baddeley, A.D. (1983). *Your Memory: A User's Guide*. Penguin, Harmondsworth.

Berloquin, P. (1980). *Games of Logic*. Unwin, London.

Brook, P., Degun, G. and Mather, M. (1975). Reality orientation, a therapy for psychogeriatric patients: a controlled study. *British Journal of Psychiatry*, **127**, 42–5.

Christensen, A.L. (1975). *Luria's Neuropsychological Investigation*. Spectrum, New York.

Cornoldi, C. (1988). Why study mnemonics? In M.M. Gruneberg, P.E. Morris and R.N. Sykes (eds.), *Practical Aspects of Memory, Vol. 2* (pp. 397–402). John Wiley and Sons, Chichester.

De Bono, E. (1979). *The Five Day Course in Thinking*. Penguin, Harmondsworth.

Folsom, J.C. (1967). Intensive hospital therapy of geriatric patients. *Current Psychiatric Therapies*, **7**, 209–15.

Folsom, J.C. (1968). Reality orientation for the elderly mental patient. *Journal of Geriatric Psychiatry*, **1**, 291–307.

Gadzella, B.M., Goldston, J.T. and Zimmerman, M.L. (1987). Effectiveness of exposure to study techniques on college students' perceptions. *Journal of Educational Research*, **71**, 26–30.

Glasgow, R.E., Zeiss, R.A., Barrera, M. and Lewinsohn, P.M. (1977). Case studies on remediating memory deficits in brain damaged individuals. *Journal of Consulting and Clinical Psychology*, **33**, 1049–54.

Godfrey, H.P.D. and Knight, R.G. (1985). Cognitive rehabilitation and memory functioning in amnesic alcoholics. *Journal of Consulting and Clinical Psychology*, **53**, 555–7.

Goldstein, G., Turner, S.M., Holzman, A., Kanagy, M., Elmore, S. and Barry, K. (1982). An evaluation of reality orientation therapy. *Journal of Behavioral Assessment*, **4**, 165–78.

Greene, J.G. (1984). The evaluation of reality orientation. In I. Hanley and J. Hodge (eds.), *Psychological Approaches to the Care of the Elderly* (pp. 192–212). Croom Helm. London.

Greene, J.G., Timbury, G.C., Smith, R. and Gardiner, M. (1983). Reality orientation with elderly patients in the community: an empirical evaluation. *Age and Ageing*, **12**, 38–43.

Hanley, I.G. (1980). Optimism or pessimism: An examination of reality orientation procedures in the management of dementia. Paper presented at the *British Psychological Society Annual Conference*, Aberdeen.

Hanley, I.G. (1981). The use of signposts and active training to modify ward disorientation in elderly patients. *Journal of Behaviour Therapy and Experimental Psychiatry*, **12**, 241–47.

Hanley, I.G. (1986). Reality orientation in the care of the elderly person with dementia – three case studies. In I. Hanley and M. Gilhooly (eds.), *Psychological Therapies for the Elderly*. London: Croom Helm.

Harley, I.G., McGuire, R.J. and Boyd, W.D. (1981) Reality orientation and dementia: a controlled trial of two approaches. *British Journal of Psychiatry*, **138**, 10–14.

Harris, J.E. (1980). We have ways of helping you remember. *Concord: The British Journal of the British Association for Service to the Elderly*, **17**, 21–7.

Hart, J. and Fleming, R. (1985). An experimental evaluation of a modified reality orientation therapy. *Clinical Gerontologist*, **3**, 35–44.

Herrmann, D., Rea, A. and Andrzejewski, S. (1988). The need for a new approach to memory training. In M.M. Gruneberg, P.E. Morris and R.N. Sykes (eds.), *Practical Aspects of Memory, Vol.* 2, (pp. 415–20). John Wiley and Sons; Chichester.

Higbee, K.L. (1981). What do college students get from a memory improvement course? Paper presented at April meeting of the Eastern Psychological Association, New York City.

Hogstel, M.O. (1979). Use of reality orientation with ageing confused patients. *Nursing Research*, **28**, 161–5.

Holden, U.P. and Sinebruchow, A. (1978). Reality orientation therapy: a study investigating the value of this therapy in the rehabilitation of elderly people. *Age and Ageing*, **7**, 83–90.

Holden, U.P. and Woods, R.T. (1982). *Reality Orientation: Psychological Approaches to the Confused Elderly.* Churchill Livingstone, London.

Johnson, C.M., McLaren, S.M. and McPherson, F. (1981). The comparative effectiveness of three versions of classroom reality orientation. *Age and Ageing*, **10**, 33–5.

Kapur, N. and Pearson, D. (1983). Memory symptoms and memory performance of neurological patients. *British Journal of Psychology*, **74**, 409–15.

Knight, R.G. and Godfrey, H.P.D. (1984). Reliability and validity of a scale for rating memory impairment in hospitalised amnesics. *Journal of Consulting and Clinical Psychology*, **52**, 769–73.

Lapp, D. (1983). Commitment: The essential ingredient in memory training. *Clinical Gerontologist*, **2**, 58–60.

Leng, N.R.C. and Parkin, A.J. (1988) Amnesic patients can benefit from instructions to use imagery: evidence against the cognitive mediation hypothesis. *Cortex*, **24**, 33–9.

McCartney, S.M. (1984). *Spatial orientation training in hospitalised patients with dementia.* Dissertation for the Diploma in Clinical Psychology, British Psychological Society, Leicester.

McDonald, M.L., and Settin, J.M. (1978). Reality orientation versus sheltered workshops as treatment for the institutionalised ageing. *Journal of Gerontology*, **33**, 416–21.

Merchant, M. and Saxby, P. (1981). Reality orientation: A way forward. *Nursing Times*, **77**, 33, 1442–5.

Randt, C.T., Brown, E.R. and Osbourne, D.P. (1980) A memory test for longitudinal measurement of mild to moderate deficits. *Clinical Neuropsychology*, **2**, 184–94.

Raven, J.C. (1960). *Guide to the Standard Progressive Matrices.* Lewis and Co. London.

Rusch, F.R. and Kazdin, A.E. (1981). Toward a methodology of withdrawal designs for the assessment of response maintenance. *Journal of Applied Behavior Analysis*, **14**, 131–40.

Voelkel, D. (1978). A study of reality orientation and resocialization groups with confused elderly. *Journal of Gerontological Nursing*, **4**, 3–18.

Wechsler, D. (1945) A standardised memory scale for clinical use. *Journal of Psychology*, **19**, 87–95.

Wilson, B.a. and Moffat, N.J. (1984a) *Clinical Management of Memory Problems*, Croom Helm, London.

Wilson, B.A. and Moffat, N.J. (1984b) Rehabilitation of memory for everyday life. in *Everyday Memory: Actions and Absent Mindedness*, eds, J. Harris and P. Morris, Academic Press, London.

Wilson, B., Cockburn, J. and Baddeley, A.D. (1985). *The Rivermead Behavioural Memory Test Manual*. Thames Valley Test Company, 7–9 The Green, Flempton, Bury St Edmunds, Suffolk.

Wing, A. and West, G. (1973). *Evans' Attainment Tests*. Evans Brothers; London.

Woods, R.T. (1979). Reality orientation and staff attention: A controlled study. *British Journal of Psychology*, **134**, 502–7.

Woods, R.T. (1983). Specificity of learning in reality orientation sessions: A single case study. *Behaviour Research and Therapy*, **21**, 173–5.

Yesavage, J.A. (1982). Degree of dementia and improvement with memory training. *Clinical Gerontologist*, **1**, 77–81.

Zarit, S.H. (1979). Helping an ageing patient to cope with memory problems. *Geriatrics*, April, 82–90.

Zarit, S.H., Zarit, J.M. and Reever, K.E. (1982). Memory training for severe memory loss: effects on senile dementia patients and their families. *Gerontologist*, **22**, 373–7.

# Chapter 10

# Self-help groups
## DEBORAH WEARING

### INTRODUCTION

As recently as 1980 America had hardly any services for brain-injured people. Then one night that year Marilyn Price Spivack, the mother of a young head-injured girl for whom there was no appropriate treatment centre, had a meeting in her home with some leading clinicians and set up the National Head Injury Foundation. The NHIF started talking to Congress and setting up a network of self-help groups all over America. The joining together of academics, clinicians and families became a powerful force. They all wanted the same things – a better understanding of brain and behaviour, more effective therapy to restore function and continuing support services.

A decade on, this powerful user-led lobby has had a remarkable effect. The USA now has around 600 brain-injury rehabilitaton programmes. They still have a long way to go – there is virtually no appropriate long-term residential care; rehabilitation programmes are generally far too short; and people with severe behaviour problems have very few units open to them. But the vast amount that has been achieved has been largely due to this self-help movement. The impetus comes from the real needs of brain-injured people.

The NHIF model is one which could be applied anywhere in the world.

Neuroscience is one of the most exciting areas of research right now. The frontiers of understanding of brain structures, neural networks, neurochemistry, cognition and behaviour are constantly being pushed outwards. Yet the advances in knowledge are not necessarily being translated into clinical work. In other words, the patients are at the bottom of the pile. The forum of a self-help group gives everyone a voice. The focus is on practical application. The knowledge of researchers, clinicians and families is mutually enriched. That consensus then has a more powerful and effective voice with clearer objectives.

A self-help group can be a few people meeting in someone's kitchen for a cup of tea, or it can be a throng in a hospital common room. It can be somewhere to get things off your chest where everyone will know what you are talking about, or where for once you are not the only one who can't remember how they got there that evening. It can be a teaching group, a research sample, a campaign team, or a melting pot where scientists, clinicians and families merge ideas. It can even develop care facilities of its own. But, most of all, it is a platform where members have a voice and where community representatives come to address this specific need.

It should be easy to make a convincing case. In Britain most severe brain injury happens to young men aged 17–22 (Medical Disability Society, 1988) with all their lives before them. The right kind of treatment and support applied by staff with the appropriate expertise over a long enough period can have remarkably good results. There is compelling evidence for the efficacy of cognitive remediation, but not much of it, and largely restricted to single case studies. A group could encourage brain injury units to measure results and conduct long-term follow up studies. Even within a self-help group there might nestle a wealth of data: relatives will have observed things over long exposure that neuropsychological test batteries would not be sensitive to. As they become more informed about brain function they may have valuable contributions to make, through psychologists in the group, to the literature.

One important reason for the scarcity of decent brain injury services in most countries is simply that there has not been a strong representative body making a convincing case for resources. Someone has to wave the banner.

In Britain the 1990 National Health Service and Community Care Act (1990) heralds changes mooted in a Government White Paper, *Working for Patients* (Department of Health Report, 1989) which asserts that user groups should be consulted in service planning and provision. What stronger argument for mustering forces?

Affiliation to a national charity such as AMNASS (The Amnesia Association) or HEADWAY (The National Head Injuries Association) plugs a local group into back-up advice, literature, newsletters, events and information and can represent local views in national lobbying.

The broader the consensus, the stronger the voice. That is why AMNASS led an initiative to persuade all the British brain injury charities to join a consortium in order to work together on common issues such as lobbying, public relations and dissemination of information.

But if all that sounds too daunting, start with the cup of tea in the kitchen and see how you get on.

## THE NEED FOR SELF-HELP GROUPS

### The practical and psycho-social effects of brain injury

Families are often struck by the marked contrast between the frenetic activity surrounding the crisis of illness or head injury, when a hospital springs into action with emergency lights flashing, and then the long haul afterwards when the brain-injured person and the family may be left largely to their own devices. At first the remit was simple: to save life. As soon as the brief gets complicated, it can seem to the family as though the hospital loses interest. As a BBC TV 'Brass Tacks' documentary on brain injury (1988) put it, 'If a life is worth saving, it has to be made worth living.' Presented with someone displaying a variety of cognitive, functional and behavioural deficits, a recovery curve that is impossible to plot and no co-ordinated brain injury service, hospitals tend to discharge and the family can be cast adrift with little preparation and back-up. Ironically, the family is typically excluded in the hospital: waiting in the corridor during the Consultant's rounds, confined to visiting hours. The doctor is usually a neurologist, neurosurgeon or general physician, whose knowledge may not extend beyond the brain tissue to the consequences of damage and the possibilities of rehabilitation. It is not enough to tell the families about the neuropathology. They need to know its possible effects and how to help.

Yet, on discharge, the family may assume all responsibility overnight. This comes hard on the heels of inevitable shock, grief and major life changes, or before these have fully registered.

Resources devoted to the support of brain-injured families in the long term are meagre the world over. Appropriate care for those without families is almost non-existent. In the Los Angeles Head Injury Survey (Jacobs, 1988) Jacobs reported that families assume most of the responsibility of care for want of any alternative. He reported that 'during the project we typically received 5–10 impassioned calls per week from families who cannot find needed services for their survivor and were on the verge of breaking up, putting the person in an institution, or taking some other drastic action'. The report also revealed that in 36.6% of cases examined (n=142) the survivor had to be continuously supervised by a family member, and that half of these carers had had to give up their job or full-time education in order to do so.

According to the *National Directory of Head Injury Rehabilitation Services* published by the National Head Injury Foundation (1988), the USA has very few life-long residential units although 'some facilities which have had experience of other handicapped populations are beginning to explore this possibility'; and only a small number of units are prepared to handle patients who exhibit destructive or sexual behaviour. To date Britain too has virtually none. People requiring these special units are randomly placed in homes for the mentally or physically handicapped, mentally ill or psycho-geriatric.

Most brain injury victims are young and there are too many survivors to be ignored. In a typical UK Health District, population 250,000, there are 250–375 people with chronic disability from a severe brain injury at any one time (Medical Disability Society, 1988).

Traditionally, physical disability is the first to get attention. Why? Certainly it is more obvious and perhaps easier to deal with. But given a choice over the ability to walk or the ability to think, I know which I would choose.

If anyone needs convincing, the literature makes plain

that cognitive, memory and behavioural functioning have the most important bearing on whether or not someone can go home, live independently, go back to work or school. A national survey by Al Condeluci (1985) for the National Head Injury Foundation showed that these deficits are 'the most disabling consequences of head injury'. See how society reacts to disability? Ramps and wide supermarket aisles are easy. But what happens to the person who cannot find their way to the shops, and would not know what to buy if they got there?

Someone may have preserved skills and remain intellectually intact and lucid, and with unimpaired speech. But if they behave in a disinhibited, aggressive or sexually inappropriate way, or if they forget everything after half-an-hour, how many places and people will tolerate them? Relatives of memory-impaired people often complain that they are met with very little comprehension of their situation, especially when the impairment is very selective and the person presents normally.

If we take Descartes' axiom 'I think therefore I am', we can deduce that a thinking disorder can play havoc with being. The reality behind deficits in memory, attention, emotion and behaviour is that some organic insult or injury can damage the mechanism of the mind so that the self is no longer in control. The self may no longer know itself or its surroundings. Memory loss can plunder your very autobiography, rub out new experience as it occurs, leaving the victim stranded in a vacuum with no yesterdays to explain the todays. Some outsiders whimsically envy the amnesiac, his ability to live only in the present.* But if the present is not rooted in a past, the present can be blotted out by a bewilderment and confusion which is only alleviated by engaging attention in pursuit of some procedural skill, in the course of which the amnesiac forgets his amnesia.

The experience of amnesia calls into question the whole concept of consciousness as well as self. My husband Clive, for example, ascribes his virtually total anterograde amnesia to 'unconsciousness'. The sensation of having no memory

---

* The masculine pronoun is used in this chapter for ease of expression and because most brain-injured people are male.

prior to the current 30 seconds is akin to the moment of waking. Therefore he is constantly (even on the point of sleep) shocked by the extraordinary phenomenon of having a moment ago woken up, yet being perhaps fully clothed and in the middle of something. How peculiar to suddenly wake up before a near-empty plate with no recollection of any but the current mouthful. When the plate is empty he has no *knowledge* of having eaten, but the bemusing and incontrovertible evidence of a full stomach and the empty plate.

Finding himself each minute suddenly awake in this way is so momentous that he is compelled to record it. He writes an ever-repeating series of entries in his diary: '3.05 p.m. – AWAKE FIRST TIME'. (He generally writes in capital letters, as he did when transcribing text as a musicologist, to mark the importance of legibility of each word.) Faced with previous recordings of awakening in his own handwriting covering every page of his diary (there is very little else of more significance to write), Clive refuses to accept that they were written when conscious. 'I have no knowledge of writing that,' he insists. 'It's different now. I'm properly awake. I wasn't conscious when I wrote that. It has nothing to do with me. *Consciousness has to involve me.*'

The dependency that memory impairment brings can force someone to regress to childlike behaviour – even if this is not provoked directly by organic damage. This brings its own problems. The ignominy of role reversal in needing guidance from your small child causes unhappiness to both. It can happen that the carer, especially a parent, reinforces dependency unwittingly through an understandably over-developed protective role. The offspring then is less able to take risks and go it alone. This is born out by I.V. Thomsen's (1984) 10–15 year follow-up study where she gives the reason for the increased number of people living independently at second follow-up as 'death of parents'. The inference must be that they might have lived independently sooner.

Perhaps the hardest thing for families to bear is be-havioural and personality disturbance. Various follow-up studies indicate that disorders such as irritability and emo-tional lability actually *increase* over time. This is likely to be due to the subsidence of other disorders leading to increased insight, and the cumulative distress at chronic disability. Another strong argument for cognitive, functional and behavioural rehabilitation in the early years.

In Britain, until now, rehabilitation for the mental disorders from brain injury have been available in only a handful of centres. Yet this country has arguably some of the most eminent neuropsychologists and neuropsychiatrists in the world. Most of their pioneering work goes on in the research laboratory, not in clinical settings. This is happily changing. The Government has plans to introduce a pilot 'model brain injury service' so that specialist treatment and care can be developed around the country.

There is a new understanding that many of the problems arising from brain injury are *not* intractable. It is proven (Eames and Wood, 1985) that appropriate rehabilitation given for long enough can make remarkable improvements, enabling some to return to employment and independent living. Rehabilitation has been dismissed by some as expensive; but costs are offset against the saving in life-long residential or other care and, of course, the returns on investment in rehabilitation are very much more than just financial.

Meanwhile, the vast majority of brain-injured people live with their families and have had no specialist rehabilitation. Many complain that there is no appropriate support in the community. It is especially difficult to provide for the special needs of brain-injured people, particularly when there are behavioural problems. So many families have told me that they cannot make use of those domiciliary care agencies that do exist because 'my wife would never learn to recognize the home visitor', or 'my husband goes beserk if people patronize him or say the wrong thing'; or, more often, 'they sent a carer to give me a break, but the carer couldn't grasp his memory problem'.

It appears that memory impairment, particularly when someone is otherwise virtually normal, is the hardest thing for the uninitiated to grasp. One mother in Manchester told me that her daughter, amnesic since an aneurysm at age 19, was to attend a day centre at the psychiatric hospital. She spent a couple of hours in discussion with the staff to make sure they understood her daughter's amnesia. After the first day she went to collect her but arrived to find that she was lost. 'Well', explained a staff member, 'we told her the way to lunch, but she never arrived.' Naturally, the poor girl had forgotten the directions almost immediately and had no idea where she was supposed to go, or why, or what she was doing there. So she found herself in the alcoholics' clinic and sat there for she knew not how long, in the expectation that somehow her mother would eventually find her. One of very many similar incidents.

A woman in Worthing had been looking after her amnesic husband for years after his head injury. She herself was chronically sick and needed a break for her own treatment, so a place was found for him in respite care. Ten days later he and two respite staff were back on the doorstep. 'We're very sorry,' explained the staff; 'we cannot cope with your husband any longer because he is aggressive.' So this sick lady was left to cope alone with him.

A frail elderly lady living alone in a sheltered flat in London now looks after her amnesic son since his herpes encephalitis. He has the bed and she sleeps on the couch. She shudders to think what might happen to him when she dies.

A young amnesic mother living with her mother and daughter in London is terrified of going out, or even of answering the door, in case she does not recognize neighbours or greets strangers. She is bored out of her mind and sees almost no one beyond the family, but says 'What is the point of going out if I don't remember it afterwards?' This lady has preserved skills and deserves rehabilitation to increase her independence, to get her back to some part-time work, and to support her in her role as mother. Her own mother needs a break from looking after the three of them.

One young man who was a law undergraduate at Cambridge when he had a cerebral haemorrhage has developed over several years an astonishingly successful use of strategies and memory aids. His system began very simply and then he built on it. This enables him to live independently and to attend college to study furniture-making – the ideal pursuit for someone amnesic. He may not freely recall how to make a particular joint but, given the environmental cues of tools and wood, he can make it. Nevertheless, at the end of the day, the only record he has of that day is notes he has taken at the time which are edited nightly and transcribed into appointments log, journal and programmed into his databank alarm watch. Even with such independence, the young man asserts with characteristic understatement that 'There is nothing good about amnesia.'

Relatives of brain-injured people the world over will find such stories only too familiar. But happily, things are changing. The UK's National Health Service and Community Care Act 1990 (Department of Health, 1990) is set to redress problems highlighted by Sir Roy Griffiths in his report to the British Government (Griffiths, 1988). He called community care 'a poor relation; everybody's distant relative, but nobody's baby'. The same might be said of brain injury as compared to other disabilities. The report saw families, friends and neighbours as a primary source of care and acknowledged that 'a failure to give proper levels of support to informal carers not only reduces their own quality of life and that of the relative or friend they care for, but is also potentially inefficient as it can lead to less personally appropriate care being offered'. The thrust of the ensuing Government White Paper (Department of Health, 1989) was towards specialist services provided by a pragmatic mix of public, private and voluntary sectors.

Let us hope that implementation of the new Act leads to better services for individuals in maximizing potential recovery, and for carers in supporting them.

The unremitting effects of memory, cognitive and behavioural disorders are very hard for families to contend with, and more so when compounded by economic pressure, a vain search for appropriate treatment, shifts in family dynamics, loss of job in order to assume the carer role, plus grief about the brain injury and losing the partner or child one knew. Some say they have lost a husband and gained a mentally disabled child.

There are practical difficulties of being responsible day and night for someone who may not know their way around the house, who might wander outside and become lost, who might forget a tap turned on or an unlit gas jet. A simple shopping trip can be highly stressful if your husband refuses to enter the shop but angrily insists on waiting outside. Will he forget what he is waiting for and wander off? You both want to use the public lavatories: can you emerge before he does? Might he leave by another exit? Imagine going up to a strange man and saying 'Excuse me, could you see if my husband is in the Gents? He has amnesia . . .'.

Then there are the deeply unsettling problems when an amnesic person does not recognize his relatives or is confused about them. One woman described to me how her husband's long retrograde amnesia would make him believe (after over twenty years of marriage) that she was just a girlfriend. Every night he would kick her out of bed for fear that they would be discovered by his parents (deceased) whom he believed to be in the next room. There were also daily rows with his 19-year-old son as he thought he was still a little boy and should not go out alone in the evening. One of many proofs that retrograde amnesia is **not** of a consistent time-span.

The stresses of living with someone – especially someone you love – who behaves so irrationally defy imagining.

There is no doubt that the hardest aspect, in the case of densely amnesic people, is the constant repetition. Some people repeat the same few comments and questions, maybe a silly joke or catchphrase, in the same tone of voice, in the same words, all the time, for the rest of their lives. The cycle of questions is usually repeated much more frequently to family members than to anyone else. Some carers develop a facility to block this out to some extent. But, to most, it is a constant and exasperating torment. The carers' threshold for this repetition and perseveration generally lowers over time. It may be this aspect alone which makes it impossible for a carer to cope at home.

So here is a group of people – brain-injured and their relatives – in very great need indeed:

1. Inadequate rehabilitation means brain-injured people may never develop the compensatory strategies and use of memory aids which could make them more independent.
2. Families cope, or fail to, largely unsupported.
3. The condition is barely understood by the wider public, or even by the medical and social services professionals

so the family's problems may be misunderstood and not appreciated.
4. Memory, cognitive and behavioural dysfunctions are devastatingly and chronically disabling, and have serious effects on a person's ability to relate to others, and are immensely difficult to live with.

Ironically, this group of people will be the least able to seek help. Care services may be unavailable for reasons given above; and carers who must always take their charge everywhere if there is no one else to deputize at home, may not be able to contemplate going to a regular carers' group. The social network of the family often falls away because a memory-impaired person may not be able to engage in normal chats and, in any case, forgets visits and perhaps forgets people. The individual may not be able to go out alone without getting lost or, with attendant behavioural problems, it may be impossible to go to social settings. So **isolation** is a very common complaint from individual and family.

But Dr Oliver Sacks once said to me. 'The remedy for grief is action.' And the remedy for isolation is getting together.

Enter the self-help group.

### Information

One of the key roles of a self-help group is to co-ordinate dissemination of information – from professionals to families, from families to professionals, from the group to health and social services, from the group to other groups and local bodies, to employers, to schools, and broadly to the general public through the media and through events.

### Carers

Dr Jonathan Miller, the neuropsychologist, opera producer and broadcaster, calls amnesia 'the carers' disease'.

The first call on information comes from families. They may be pretty confused in the early months. In the beginning doctors cannot know the full extent of brain damage, they cannot predict the prognosis, and they may not even know if the patient will live. Then once the picture begins to emerge, it may be too appalling to accept and relatives commonly experience denial, which may take several forms, neatly analysed by George Prigatano (Klonoff and Prigatano, 1987). This is functional, as a coping mechanism, and should not be dismantled too brutally; but it can be dysfunctional when families develop unrealistic expectations which put pressure on their relative, on the staff, or which interfere with teaching compensatory strategies – say, on the grounds that a diary is 'cheating'. At this time the last thing a family may see is that they have anything in common with a support group for 'disabled' people.

However, hospitals often use support group literature to give to families so that they can read about brain injury in their own time. It may contain important advice which relatives should consider from the outset, such as legal and insurance issues after an accident. Other literature explains about the brain and the effects of damage. In a state of shock and grief, it may not be possible to take in all that the doctors are saying. Having the literature and a telephone number to call someone outside the hospital gives relatives a chance to get more information. The very vocabulary may all be new. What are occipito-parietal lobes? What happens if they're damaged? What's the difference between a psychiatrist and a psychologist? A self-help group and its leaflets can go a long way to demystify brain injury.

A further advantage to be gained from understanding brain function is that families might develop a more clinical perspective, a crucial coping mechanism. Being aware of the underlying neuropathology which is causing bizarre behaviour helps to modify one's emotional response. So many relatives engage in endless and fruitless arguments with someone whose reason is impaired, or who cannot remember the facts under discussion, or who is perseverative. To some, to dismiss their spouse's statements as mentally impaired would seem like a gross betrayal. And it is impossible to change the way one relates to someone overnight, even if they become brain injured. But the difference is this: your husband hits you or does something embarrassing in public; you can either get upset and remonstrate with him, or you can say to yourself 'Ooh, he's being a bit frontal today', and engage his attention in something quiet. Information can help save carers from being reduced to a brain-injured existence themselves, trapped in an amnesic loop tape.

Leaflets can only go so far. Support groups based in hospitals tend to put relatives in touch with another family who are further down the line. They can demonstrate improvement and provide encouragement. Some hospitals see self-help groups as an important supplement to care. One rehabilitation unit in Boston, Massachusetts, employs a Family Advocate, a formal personification of this role. She is the mother of a head-injured boy, and families feel very comfortable with her since she knows exactly how they must be feeling. She acts as an intermediary between staff and families.

### Group support

The value of sharing experiences with others who have been through something similar cannot be overstated. The problems presented by memory disordered people are singular and often very hard to bear. The effects upon the carer of endless repetition, confabulation, emotional lability and behavioural disturbance are significant and sometimes insupportable. To take the repetition alone – to be forced to utter the same dialogue, perhaps verbatim, with little alteration of inflection or intonation would be a torture of Sisyphean proportions if it only lasted a day. But the cumulative effects of fielding infinitely repeated questions for years and decades with seldom any respite are colossal. Fortunately Brooks *et al.* (1986) have measured the typical lowering of the relatives' tolerance threshold in a five- to seven-year follow-up study. With this effect documented there is no excuse for neglecting to guard against it by increasing support.

Getting together with others in a group does help people to feel less isolated, less singled out for misfortune. The dread question 'Why us?' dims when you are sitting amid a roomful of people in the same boat.

Groups which concentrate almost exlusively on mutual support for carers do not suit everyone. Meetings can end up as sessions for people to vie with each other as to the awfulness of their situation, or the degree of impairment of their relative. If discussions are allowed to sink to this too frequently they could simply end up depressing everyone.

AMNASS West London branch was losing members, but resolved to 'talk less about how terrible it is, and actually *do* something'.

### People with a brain injury

By far the most acute needs come from brain injured people themselves, although the degree of their memory and cognitive impairment will determine the degree of their awareness. Many self-help groups have meetings where brain-injured people, their relatives and professionals mix. I favour those which split up so that people can get away from their carers, and vice versa. The groups which seem to work best are those which structure their time and which are designed carefully to suit the needs of members. One AMNASS group has a psychologist facilitating discussion among a group of young amnesic people. She employs various aids, including drawing. Her members may not recognize each other, or recall discussion from one meeting to the next, but they will recognize their own drawing and recapture in it the mood of the last discussion. It supplies a sense of continuity. Group meetings can also be used to introduce memory aids and strategies. Any funds the group raises might be used to purchase the more expensive electronic memory aids (or persuade manufacturers to donate them) in order for members to use.

It can be a relief to be surrounded by other people who do not recognize you either and who are as confused as you. There is no need to cover up, to half-smile at anyone and everyone in case you know them. No need to stifle the question that you may have asked a hundred times or not at all. No need to fear admitting that you have no idea whether this is London or Manchester. This is the one place where it is 'safe' to be amnesic.

There is a danger, with brain-injured people in particular, that they will not be accorded the same respect and powers of advocacy that others take for granted. They suffer particularly from patronizing voices and condescending attitudes, partly because they are so vulnerable that they need protecting, and partly because lack of knowledge and lack of memory are equated with childishness.

A group should take care to build in strong roles for amnesic people. They usually have preserved skills, so would be able to contribute to the running of the group, for example, in typing correspondence, illustrating posters, preparing refreshments and – most importantly – in determining group policy, and in making representations as far as they are able. One AMNASS group's report to the Annual General Meeting consisted chiefly of a taped speech by an amnesic member who had worked hard in preparing it with the group. It was the most powerful speech of the day.

The group might be the only place where memory-impaired people have the chance to enjoy a sense of achievement and involvement.

The Chairman of the USA's National Head Injury Foundation, in his address to their 1987 symposium, urged that giving people with a brain injury a voice 'should be the Foundation's single most important role'. Their newsletter had a column called 'First Person' written by a head-injured person. AMNASS's RECALL magazine has a similar column called 'Metamemory'.

### Clinicians and researchers

Professionals benefit from the deeper knowledge they acquire through long-term observation. The group provides more verismo than the ward or laboratory. They discover strategies which work or don't work in everyday life. The psychologist who runs an Age Concern group for carers of dementia sufferers in Exeter commented 'We frequently find that a great many carers are themselves "experts" in their particular role of caring and have a lot to teach the professionals and to give to other carers.'

The group may well provide a living research sample; in that context there is an opportunity for amnesic people and relatives to discuss fully the ethical questions surrounding any piece of research, question the methodology, and to decide if they want to take part. Professionals too have the chance to explain exactly what they are doing and where they hope the research will lead. It may be that the views of the group will lead to a modification of the research or even a rejection of the paradigm.

Some self-help groups commission their own research, usually of a practical nature. Headway Cambridge ran a project to compile a handbook describing facilities and services for head-injured people in the district. National charities usually have their own science committees responsible for clinical and research issues. The AMNASS Scientific Group, for example, convened a meeting of interested psychologists to look at the various memory assessment techniques. Then it set out to develop a comprehensive test battery which would cover every kind of memory function – selecting existing tests where appropriate and designing new ones for memory functions for which there was no good measure.

Well-resourced groups might run research funds and look at grant proposals submitted. Where there is such money I would hope that the membership would specify the research they want, rather than sitting back to wait for the research grant proposals they get. Where there isn't such money, but where a research need emerges, then the group should secure funding from one of the many charitable trusts which like research but recoil from core funding.

General Practitioners are often the clinicians most in contact with brain-injured people in the community and are worth cultivating. But they probably have the least time to attend a group's meeting or open day. Self-help groups concerned with different aspects of brain injury – aphasia, memory problems, stroke – would do well to band together to produce a brain injury information pack for GPs describing the possible conditions and giving reference sources on treatment. It should be easy to handle, clear and quick to assimilate if you want it to be used. A video (if you can get sponsorship . . . there are 48,000 GPs in Britain) gets the message across with more impact; but keep it short – say, maximum 15 minutes, and it is more likely to get watched.

## THE DEVELOPMENT OF SELF-HELP GROUPS

One of the early self-help groups to be established in Britain was the Association of Parents with Backward Children in 1946. It became known as the Royal Society for Mentally Handicapped Children and Adults, or MENCAP, and has grown from a small nucleus of enthusiastic parents, to a Society of 55,000 members. With 550 local groups and eight divisional offices it now provides homes, training centres, employment services (open and sheltered), 700 Gateway clubs (for leisure) with the involvement of 20,000 volunteers serving 40,000 members, and a great deal more.

Innovative and successful groups which came from small beginnings and which have made important contributions to the care of people with learning difficulties in Britain include the Camphill Village Trust and the Home Farm Trust where people live and work in self-sufficient, but not self-contained, communities.

Self-help groups in general were still thin on the ground in 1960 but came into their own in the 1970s when consumer movements and the media were encouraging the participation of the critical consumer. The aims of groups concerned with brain injury worldwide are similar – the result of common problems. They are broadly:

1. To provide support for patients and their families within a social network of people who understand the nature of the problem;
2. To inform patients and their families about the after-effects of injury and ways of dealing with them;
3. To access services in the community which will alleviate the difficulties of care;
4. To press for, and possibly to create, better rehabilitation, care and support services;
5. To increase public awareness of the problems;
6. To learn more about the condition through long-term liaison between families and professionals;
7. To promote research advancing knowledge about the disorders and improved rehabilitation techniques.

During the 1980s the number of self-help groups serving disabilities has proliferated, and the voluntary sector, with encouragement from government, has become very much more professional, now working in association with the public and private sectors.

The two main groups for people with non-dementing memory problems are AMNASS and Headway, and are outlined here.

### AMNASS, The Amnesia Association

I founded AMNASS with Dr Barbara Wilson in 1986. I founded it when I found that there were no services for my husband, Clive, after he contracted herpes encephalitis in 1985 aged 47. He was admitted to a major London teaching hospital and has remained there ever since, for seven months on a general ward, and then on a psychiatric ward. Barbara Wilson had seen many other people for whom there were no services so we joined forces to do something about it. We used Dr Jonathan Miller's TV documentary about Clive as our launching pad. That film, 'Prisoner of Consciousness' was seen in over 20 countries and led to much more media coverage.

AMNASS's objectives are:

1. To give support and information to sufferers and families;
2. To promote the interests of memory-impaired people;
3. To urge for provision of appropriate rehabilitation and care facilities;
4. To offer information, seminars and workshops to professionals;
5. To encourage research.

The newsletter, RECALL, is AMNASS's principal means of communication. It carries news, views and advice to a mixed audience of families and professionals on many issues, from neuroscience and how a virus might cross the blood/brain barrier, to income support and attendance allowance.

AMNASS has generated a strong flow of media interest in amnesia and the problems it brings – something which was scarcely known about before, even within the medical and paramedical professions. Increasing public awareness is preparing the ground for change.

The Association is actively engaged in representing the

needs of its members to central and local government and to care agencies who may suddenly find themselves with a memory-impaired patient and no idea how to respond.

The AMNASS Scientific Group numbers some of the country's leading neuropsychologists and neuropsychiatrists, advising on all aspects of clinical work, individual queries, in-house literature, training and research. It runs residential workshops combining theory and practical sessions. An AMNASS workshop typically covers causes and psychological theories, an overview of current knowledge, assessment techniques, clinical aspects and management.

A small but growing number of local groups provides an important forum, or haven, for members.

### Headway: The National Head Injuries Association

Headway was founded in the UK in 1979 by Reg Talbott, previously a social worker. Local branches have evolved in different ways, according to the direction taken by members. Some may be active in the broader aims of Headway, such as the prevention of head injury, promoting the concept of rehabilitation and community care for head-injured people, or forging links with hospitals.

A number of Headway branches have followed the example of Roger Fitzsimmons, a speech therapist who co-ordinates the branch at Gloucester. He started the first Headway House. This is a day centre for head-injured people to come to regularly. Here they can get involved with real occupations, learn new skills, practise old ones. It gives them an all-important sense of self-worth and gets them out of the house. Meanwhile carers have a break to go out shopping or have some precious time to themselves. Staffing is largely voluntary at these centres, but may well be attached to a hospital and be supervised by clinicians there. Equipment and furnishings are, it is hoped, donated by traders in the local community.

More and more Headway Houses are springing up. Meanwhile they are setting off on an ambitious new venture. They have teamed up with the Disabled Housing Trust to develop Headway Rehabilitation Centres. The first is set to open in Milton Keynes in 1991 and a second is planned for Leeds where there happens to be one of only a couple of the UK's University rehabilitation departments.

Headway, like AMNASS, runs conferences for clinicians and researchers and actively encourages research. In one study it acted as a control group. There will always be hazards with questionnaire, self-reporting surveys; but a Headway carer is probably going to give more reliable answers than many uninitiated clinicians. With its many hundreds of members it is probably the most valuable living databank on brain injury in the country.

There are a number of charities for specific disorders associated with brain injury in the UK and these are listed at the end of the chapter. Whether a memory disorder arises from anoxia during cardiac arrest, or from a tumour, so that it develops at a different rate, the effects and the problems will ultimately be similar. Just as each self-help group can grow to support the specific needs of its own members, so different groups will have important issues in common. It makes sense to seek out other groups representing brain-injured people and collaborating with them on, say, lobbying local authorities, public awareness campaigns, education and information services, placing media stories and so on. If you have a particularly important speaker, share the event with other charities: the speaker is more impressed by the numbers and is more likely to take you seriously, the talk is of wider benefit, and you are likely to get more publicity. Several groups together might share a 'drop-in' advice centre, a telephone counselling service, TV/radio helplines, and the costs of producing information packs.

The UK's national brain-injury charities are planning to associate in this way in a consortium principally for lobbying and public awareness purposes. There is no reason why local groups should not do the same.

A close working relationship across self-help groups can only benefit members and improve effectiveness through a wider information base and by giving them a stronger, more representative voice.

## STARTING AND RUNNING A GROUP

### Setting up

The impetus for starting a group often comes from carers. When impotent to help their injured relative they may either be preoccupied with the hard grind of caring, or they may choose to get involved with the general cause. Running or participating in a group gives scope to step out of the passive role and take control of the situation. The close involvement of professionals, especially for an emergent group, is helpful as they may be better placed to provide premises and administrative back-up, in addition to giving technical and clinical advice.

The nucleus membership wanting to start a group might find these guidelines helpful.

First things first: do not re-invent the wheel! Find out whether there is a self-help support team in your area. In Britain the National Council for Voluntary Organizations (NCVO) will put you in touch with one. Self-help support teams are a marvellous band of people offering local knowledge, a resource base and encouragement (or devil's advocacy, whichever you appear to need). They may help you set up your first meeting, talking to their media contacts and lending their photocopier and mailing lists. Some even make a grant towards setting up expenses. They usually attend the inaugural meeting and talk to those present about what a group might do or be. Then they can help you develop afterwards – networking with other groups and with health and social services, accessing information, resources, grants, speakers.

Just this networking exercise through the Support Team goes a long way towards making brain injury and memory problems more widely understood by the community.

Here is a basic checklist of preparations for your inaugural meeting:

Fix a time and venue which is easily accessible from transport and by wheelchair, and fairly large in case your publicity is effective. Then contact all interested parties. Professionals should check through records and contact former patients. Circulate GPs, social workers, health visitors, rehabilitation centres, nursing and special homes, day centres and special schools; send them posters and ask them to contact families they know of. Notices can be displayed in libraries and GP surgeries. Make announcements through the local media. Most local radio stations have a community service. Get on the air – a clinician and a family member make a good double act. Prepare a single sheet giving a brief statement of the purpose of forming the group, the range of membership (e.g. precisely which disability interest, families, friends, clinicians, social workers, community workers, volunteers . . .), the date, time and place.

At the first meeting a chairman should outline an agenda so that time is spent in productive discussion of people's interests, and what they would like from a group. Perhaps not everyone will have a chance to – or want to – speak, so distribute a questionnaire so that you have a record of names and addresses, and so that people have a chance to express their views.

It may be that the group naturally splits into local sub-groups, or sections serving different needs. At the outset members should explore their own objectives and agree priorities. Programme time for a social gathering afterwards so that the important business of getting to know each other can begin. With the degree of social isolation among brain injured families, social opportunities are highly valued.

The optimal size of a group depends on its purpose. If the primary aim is mutual support, then up to a dozen people in someone's front room might be right. With that aim, it is probably more important to try to match like with like. When Janis Morris was running the King's Fund 'Head Injury Case Management Study' she advocated that groups match people with others whose circumstances are as similar as possible, and keeping the group small in size. She suggested that group members would be more likely to form strong bonds with each other if they are of similar age and background and contending with similar problems.

What ratio of family members to professionals works best? A Headway group, which ran for a time at London's Homerton Regional Neurological Rehabilitation Unit, folded. Members believe this was because the group was led by professionals and families never became closely enough involved. AMNASS has found that groups work best when the special contribution that each member can bring is recognized and used.

Then there is the sheerly practical question of attending meetings. People caring at home on a restricted income may find long journeys difficult or out of the question. Public transport may not be an option if the relative has a behavioural disorder. AMNASS Manchester has some people commuting from as far as Liverpool, while others never attend at all because they do not have transport.

### Activities

So what might a self-help group actually do? Good advice from Judy Wilson of the Nottingham Self-Help Support Team is 'Do not run before you can walk' (Wilson, 1986, 1988). The broad range of activities suggested in this chapter need not all be included in a group's manifesto; they are rather options to explore at one time or another, not necessarily all at once! It is quite important that priorities should be determined by members, and that goals should not be over-ambitious or the group might fall at the first fence.

One early goal might be to foster a working relationship with other community bodies. This way, you quickly establish a broad base of support – either for funding, services, advice or simply general goodwill, which can do a surprising amount to buoy up people who have got used to feeling misunderstood and neglected. If you develop a simple talk/ presentation which members can give to Women's Institutes, Chambers of Commerce, to schools etc, you soon multiply the number of people who have a grasp of brain injury, and who remember you next time they have to nominate a charity to receive funds. One thing about amnesia – it is so extraordinary, that people *do* remember it. Your network of support might come from:

Community Health Councils
Councils for Voluntary Service/Action
Citizen's Advice Bureaux
Social Services
Women's Groups

Religious Bodies
Related Charities, e.g. Carers' Groups, Stroke Clubs
Family Practitioner Committee
General Medical Council
The Patients' Association
The Informal Caring Support Unit, King's Fund Centre
British Legion
St John Ambulance
Youth Clubs
Schools, Colleges
Rotary Clubs/Round Tables
Chambers of Commerce
The media
Local employers (especially past employers of group members)

Every member will be in some way connected to a whole array of organizations – and there is no doubt that a personal contact is the most effective way of attracting support.

The broader the base of support, the more widely the group's interests will become known. The more goodwill and help forthcoming, the more you will be able to achieve. Today someone to listen, tomorrow a counselling service. Today a meeting place, tomorrow a day centre. How you welcome newcomers to the group is important. Have a policy, so that people don't feel excluded by a cosy clique; perhaps assign people to take newcomers under their wing.

Set some parameters from the outset. If people are going to give their home telephone numbers as 'helplines', are they prepared for the phone to ring at any time of day or night with distress calls? Are members equal to dealing with calls from brain-injured people? From family members? Will they know what advice to give? Perhaps people embarking on such an exercise would benefit from some training in counselling skills. Members might learn from other groups of their experience in offering helplines. Would they rather join up with associated charities and share a line to be manned during set hours?

If professionals have set up the group, do they wish to continue with management indefinitely, or should family members be integrated into the team?

Then there is the programme of activities. Here are some suggestions:

Run a memory group in which rehabilitation techniques can be introduced; families can try methods of generalizing learning and exchanging notes with clinicians on what works and how.

Collect a memory-aid library which members can learn to use in the group and at home.

Invite speakers from any of the organizations listed above.

Design and make posters to represent graphically the group's problem.

Get someone else to design and print your poster for nothing – say, a competition in the local newspaper, a project at a school or college art department; the guaranteed media coverage and prize-giving event should persuade a local printer to run off a batch for nothing.

Have a workshop for carers.

Run a workshop for the local hospital/University psychology/OT/speech/physiotherapy department.

Watch a video on head injury.

Go to the movies!

Have an open day for guests from the above organizations and from the media (see below for media pitfalls . . .).

Team up with psychology or other students who can be primed to take your younger members on regular outings, perhaps with access to sports and leisure facilities.

Set up a day centre, rehabilitation or a long-stay unit.

Have a barbecue.

Design/participate in research projects.

Have some workshops on relaxation techniques: meditation, massage, aromatherapy.

Learn about metabolic change after brain injury and have a talk on healthy eating.

Get your neuropsychiatrist to speak on drug therapies.

Get your neurologist to talk you through scanning techniques and EEGs

Produce your own newsletter, especially for members who cannot get to meetings.

Generate fundraising events (see below).

Lobby central and local Government through your MP and councillors.

This is just a bunch of ideas, in no particular order, to set the ball rolling!

### Fundraising

Even a small and simple group can incur expenses. The more you want to do, the more it may cost.

The very act of fundraising has a lot to recommend it – quite apart from the money it may produce. It attracts attention to the cause, and gives you a chance to get your message across. Moreover, there is no substitute for actually **doing** something: people feel useful and then more committed. The ordinary process of collecting bric-a-brac for a bazaar brings the group into contact with a growing network of allies among neighbours. Someone manning the cake stall may end up as a volunteer to the group. Get local traders to donate raffle prizes. Ask schools to do a sponsored swim, run, or knit for your group.

Then there is the other kind of sponsorship – corporate sponsorship of a project or for core funding for the group. Rootle out your experts for this. Someone's mother might be an accountant, lawyer or marketing manager. Get advice from the Self Help Support Team and from the national organization to which your group is affiliated. Do not attempt corporate sponsorship yourself without some specialist advice: you may be asking for £100 when the company could be persuaded to give you £1,000. Have very clear agreed objectives about what you want the money for.

Submissions for financial assistance should be made well in advance (absolute minimum six months for smaller amounts, longer for bigger projects). The proposal should give a clear outline of the purpose and list the promotional benefits that you are offering the sponsor in return (for example, accreditation on your promotional material). Costings should have been prepared in detail but the initial approach should probably only give an outline breakdown with the offer of a detailed costing if requested. It definitely pays to use a professional for this kind of fundraising activity.

### Media and public relations

The media can be among your most powerful allies. When a journalist asks a question, it can sometimes elicit a faster and possibly a better response than when an individual asks the same question. The media can also have a huge impact on public awareness, especially of commonly misunderstood conditions such as brain injury. But there are pitfalls . . .

What journalists want most is 'human interest' stories. To protect your highly vulnerable members, designate a tough but diplomatic and well-informed member to be 'press officer'. That person would dictate the interview conditions to the journalist – for example, to ask for 'copy approval'. This will normally be refused but you can insist on the grounds that the person to be interviewed does not have the capacity to recall the conversation afterwards, and may wish others to correct inaccurate statements. These are unique circumstances. Anyway, where else are they going to get an interviewee to talk about living with a memory disorder? Insist that the carer also be interviewed for the sake of accuracy. Make sure no information is disclosed which puts the interviewee at risk – e.g. where they hide their front door key, or their address. Try asking for a donation to the group in recompense for your trouble – set a sum according to the likely budget of the journal. Any filming must give you an appearance fee and a facility fee if it is on your premises. For filming on your premises ask to see a statement of indemnity to make sure that insurance cover is adequate.

Intervene if questioning goes too far. It is easier for the detached press officer to say 'Cut' than for the interviewee. Do not wait until an answer has been given and then say you would rather they did not print that bit. Unless you have secured copy approval, once words are uttered, they are as good as in print. On recorded radio or TV just say 'We agreed you would not ask questions on this subject.' They would have to edit that out. Any other reply and they might leave it in making the interviewee seem evasive.

Remember that the reporter is likely to sensationalize and make sure the interviewee is prepared for exaggerated headlines, quotes taken out of context, 'quotes' which are by no-one except the reporter, and maybe an unflattering photograph. Sometimes the nicer and more sympathetic the journalist seems to be, the more he or she may betray your wishes in the final story. Sure, this sounds cynical: but I write after being professionally involved with the media – local, national, international and specialist – as a press officer in widely differing fields over the last ten years, and also as the subject of a hackneyed human interest story. Believe me.

These warnings may make you wonder whether it is worth talking to the media at all. Certainly the scrutiny on something intensely personal can be very unpleasant. But the effects of making memory loss better understood are a necessary prelude to getting better services. This is compensation enough.

### Training and advice for groups

Usually shared experience is the mainstay of learning for members. But there are times when specialist help may be needed. This is not the place to detail exactly what help a group may require and advise on where to get it. One rule of thumb is: if you don't know, ask someone who does! The Self-Help Support Teams and voluntary organization councils are generally the fount of all knowledge. Another rule of thumb: if something seems difficult and laborious, find someone else to do it. Woo local colleges who can give your work to their students as projects. Or persuade local businesses to take it on as 'sponsorship in kind'. Sometimes that can have real pay-offs for both sides. Lowe Howard Spink, the advertising agency which ran a poster campaign in the London Underground for AMNASS completely free of charge, won a special award for it in *Campaign* magazine. Cultivate the local radio chatshow host – despite the warnings of the previous section – so that, when you are stuck for help or advice, you can go on air and appeal for what you need.

Finally, if members actually want to acquire some new skill to enable them to run the group more effectively, then take a look at the training programmes offered by various voluntary organizations, often free or very cheap. You can polish up your counselling or public speaking skills, learn about special needs housing, the NHS Community Care

Bill, disability benefits, or even . . . how to work with the media!

## CONCLUSION

All I have to say in conclusion is . . . 'Go for it!'

## REFERENCES

Brooks, D.N., Campsie, L., Symington, C., *et al.* (1986) The five year outcome of severe blunt head injury: A relative's view. *Journal of Neurology, Neurosurgery and Psychiatry*, **49**, 764–70.

Condeluci, A. (1985) *National Head Injury Survey*. National Head Injury Foundation, Washington D.C.

Department of Health Report (1989) *Working for Patients*. HMSO, London.

Department of Health (1990) *The National Health Service and Community Care Act*. HMSO, London.

Eames, P. and Wood, R. (1985) Rehabilitation after severe brain injury: A follow-up study of a behaviour modification approach. *Journal of Neurology, Neurosurgery and Psychiatry*, **48**, 137–40.

Griffiths, R. (1988) *Community Care: Agenda for Action*. HMSO, London.

Jacobs, H.E. (1988) The Los Angeles head injury survey: Procedures and initial findings. *Archives Physical Medicine and Rehabilitation*, **69**, 425–31.

Klonoff, P. and Prigatano, G.P. (1987) Reactions of family members and clinical intervention after traumatic brain injury. In M. Ylvisaker and E.M.R. Gobble (eds.) *Community Re-Entry for Head Injured Adults*. College-Hill, USA.

Medical Disability Society (1988) *The Management of Traumatic Brain Injury*. Development Trust for the Young Disabled, London.

National Head Injury Foundation (1988) *National Directory of Head Injury Rehabilitation Services*, Washington D.C.

Thomsen I.V. (1984) Late outcome of very severe blunt head trauma: A 10–15 year second follow-up. *Journal of Neurology, Neurosurgery and Psychiatry*, **47**, 260–8.

Wilson, J. (1986) *Self-help groups*. Longman, Harlow.

Wilson, J. (1988) *Caring together – guide-lines for carers' self-help groups*. Kings Fund Centre, London.

## USEFUL ADDRESSES

AMNASS – The Amnesia Association
St Charles' Hospital
Exmoor Street

London W10 6DZ
Tel. 081–969 0796

HEADWAY – The National Head Injuries Association
7 King Edward Court
King Edward Street
Nottingham NG1 1EW
Tel. 0602 240800
Fax. 0602 240432

ADA – Action for Dysphasic Adults
Canterbury House
1 Royal Street
London SE1 7LL
Tel. 071–261 9572

CHSA – Chest Heart and Stroke Association
CHSA House
Whitecross Street
London EC1Y 8JJ
Tel. 071–490 7999

MENCAP National Centre
123 Golden Lane
London EC1Y 0RT
Tel. 071–253 9433

Age Concern England
Bernard Sunley House
60 Pitcairn Rd
Mitcham
Surrey CR4 3LL
Tel. 081–640 5431

Carers' National Association
29 Chilworth Mews
London W2 3RG
Tel. 071–723 8130

King's Fund Informal Caring Support Programme
King's Fund Centre
126 Albert Street
London NW1 7NF
Tel. 071–267 6111

NCVO – National Council for Voluntary Organisations
26 Bedford Square
London WC1B 3HU
Tel. 071–636 4066

Patients' Association
18 Victoria Park Square
London E2 9PF
Tel. 081–981 5676

St John Ambulance
1 Grosvenor Crescent
London SW1X 7EF
Tel. 071–235 5231

Charities' Aid Foundation
48 Pembury Rd
Tonbridge, Kent TN9 2JD
Tel. 0732 356323

# Author index

# Subject index

External aids
  see also Memory diaries
    and aids
    62, 64, 66, 68, 70, 72, 94–96,
    97, 99, 102, 112, 132, 135, 137,
    148, 149, 254, 264
Expanded rehearsal, see
  Distribution of practice
Experimental psychology and
  experimental psychologists
  see also Psychology
    61, 165, 180, 183

Face–name association
  procedure 101, 138, 139
Face recognition 141, 176
Fading 148, 150
Familiarity 9, 34, 39, 221
Family carers and relatives 37,
    87, 95, 97, 98, 100, 108, 126,
    128, 150, 248, 249, 274, 275, 276,
    277, 278, 280, 282, 283, 286, 291,
    294, 295, 297
Fatigue 225
Feedback 87, 93, 112, 113, 167,
    170, 172, 173, 217, 229, 230, 268
Feeling of knowing 164
First letter mnemonic 63, 64,
    139, 151
Fitzsimmons, Roger 292
Flexibility 156, 172, 182, 184
Forgetting, see Memory
  problems
Forgetting curve 23
Free recall
  see also Recall
    8, 9, 10, 12, 122, 162, 164,
    193, 204
Frontal lobes (damage and
  function) 20, 34, 52, 140, 165,
    191, 217, 218, 224, 230, 233,
    266, 286
Functional communication
  skills 51

Functional skills 216, 219,
    233, 234

GABA 191, 192, 202, 203, 205
Games of logic 254
General principles (Guidelines)
    122–123
Glutamate 191
Generalization 4, 16, 27, 66, 90,
    91, 104, 114, 143, 149–51, 173,
    174, 176, 177, 183, 229, 236, 237,
    238, 246, 247, 248, 249, 251
Goal(s) 40, 54, 127, 131, 144, 147,
    232, 296
Gollin pictures 51

Halstead–Reitan 162, 174, 175
Head injury and head injured
  people
  see also Brain injury
    23, 34, 35, 36, 47, 51, 83, 87,
    88, 95, 97, 101, 103, 114, 120,
    121, 128, 134, 137, 139, 140,
    148, 157, 166, 173, 174, 175,
    176, 177, 190, 217, 219, 225,
    231, 233, 237, 244, 252, 261,
    263, 266, 269, 274, 276, 286,
    292, 298
Head injury case management
  study 295
Headway 275, 289, 291, 292, 293,
    295, 303
Hewlett–Packard (85), 163, 164
HIV 120, 127
Holden communication
  scale 247
Huntington's Disease 111, 112,
    191, 192, 202, 204, 205
Hyoscine/scopolamine 192,
    193, 195

IBM machines 154, 178, 181
Iconic memory 6

*Subject index*